FUNDAMENTALS of NEUROLOGICAL DIAGNOSIS

2

Bertha Chioma Ekeh
B Med Pharm, MBBS, FMCP (Neuro)

All the radiological images were selected with permission from
The unpublished collection of images by
Dr Nnenna Nkem Nwafor (MBBS, FWACS)
Consultant Radiologist:
University of Uyo Teaching Hospital/Ibom Specialist Hospital
Uyo
Nigeria

Front cover image culled from http://factsforkids.net/brain-facts-kids-top-15-mind-blowing-facts-human-brain-2/

Copyright © 2018 Bertha Chioma Ekeh

All rights reserved.

ISBN 1983888427
ISBN-13: 978 1983888427

First Edition

DEDICATION

TO

THE ALMIGHTY GOD FROM WHOM ALL KNOWLEDGE COME FROM

My Beloved Nephews and Nieces:

Chiagoziem
Chizitere
Amarachukwu
Akachukwu
Ikenna
Eziuche
Chisom
Joshua

You are a major part of my blessings

ACKNOWLEDGEMENTS

I hereby acknowledge my late parents Lawrence and Celina Ekeh (Great teachers themselves) for imparting in me the love and passion for teaching.

To my siblings:
Anie, Agatha, Loretta, Izuchi and Emerson
Thank you for all your love and support.

To my beloved friends:
Ugochi, Amaka, Aleruchi, Calista, Ugochukwu, Edna, Ngozi, Esther and Sylvia
Thank you for believing in me all these years

To Maryann and her sons John and Enoch
Thank you for providing me with a wonderful environment

I am indebted to Dr Ifeanyi Onwuezobe and Dr Franklin Dike for spending valuable time to proof read this book.

PREFACE

To ensure that one life breathed easier just because you lived: that is to have achieved

Ralph Waldo Emerson

The importance of good history and physical examination with proper interpretation being adequate for neurological diagnosis in as much as 90% of cases cannot be overemphasized. Investigations however are essential for collaboration with or confirmation of the clinical diagnosis. Recent advances in scientific technology have increased the physician's armamentarium in investigative modalities. The advent of these sophisticated modalities (neuro imaging techniques, biochemical and gene studies) for the investigation of neurological disorders has caused an overreliance on these investigations *alone* for diagnosis. Neurologists with access to these investigations are usually tempted to substitute them for clinical acumen. This practice should be avoided as they certainly do not guarantee the diagnosis in neurological patients. The aim of the neurologist is to arrive at a final diagnosis by the intelligent analysis of the clinical data aided by the *least number of investigations*. In essence, clinical diagnosis should always precede and guide the investigations. Hence, the practice of sending patients with neurological symptoms for a barrage of expensive investigations whose results all come out normal is particularly improper and ostentatious especially in poor resource settings where healthcare is hampered by poor funds (being mostly paid for out of pocket). In fact, spending a large portion of or all of the available funds on unnecessary investigations is ostentatious and may actually be unethical.

In some cases, physicians carry out these numerous but mostly irrelevant investigations in order to satisfy their curiosity.

Once again, this reason is not tenable because the essence of investigations should be based largely on therapeutic and prognostic considerations not on the physician's curiosity.

Furthermore some patients insist on sophisticated investigations to allay their fear of a more sinister diagnosis and doctors are forced to comply. In such a scenario, the physician owes it to the patient to educate him on his symptoms, the essential investigations and expected results. It is not always good judgment to succumb to all the patient's whims and caprices.

Noteworthy is that the African patient is apt to believe in the supernatural causes of diseases (especially neurological disorders like stroke, epilepsy, movement disorders and dementia). These apparently normal results lend some credibility to the socio-cultural beliefs which impact the health seeking behaviour, choice of treatment modality (orthodox, spiritual or traditional herbs), compliance to medications and ultimately the eventual outcome. In view of the above, it is pertinent to have a thorough clinical evaluation, localize the lesion, make a clinical diagnosis or narrow down the differential diagnosis before requesting investigations. This book 'Fundamentals of Neurological Diagnosis' gives a *simplified step wise approach* to the diagnosis of Neurological disorders. The first part is a brief anatomy of the nervous system; the second part is a guide to the localization of lesions while the third part details the basic investigations of the central nervous system. It is my utmost desire that by the virtue of this book **'Fundamentals of Neurological Diagnosis'** some persons will breathe easier in Neurological Diagnosis.

Dr Bertha C Ekeh

REVIEWS

'I actually sought out a book like this during my early clinical years, and unable to find one had no option but to face the Neurology section of Hutchison's clinical methods head on. I think the writer's penchant for teaching rubbed off a lot in the writing style, and she actually succeeds in impressing upon her readers the essential take home points. Most importantly, diagnosis in neurology requires a systematic approach on a foundation of basic neuroscience, and secondly localization is key.

It is definitely worth every second!'

Franklin O Dike
MBBCh, FWACP (Int. Med-Neuro)

I think I can give my thoughts on the book with the title 'Fundamentals of Neurological Diagnosis'. This is because; I had the rare priviledge of proof reading it.
I can say for sure, that the book is what the reader needs as a key to opening the complex door leading to the diagnosis of both common and some rare neurologic disorders. It will be of immense help to students and specialists in the field of medicine.

IFEANYI A. ONWUEZOBE
MBBCH, M.SC, M.PH, FMCPATH (NIG), FCPATH ECSA.

CONTENT

		Acknowledgments	I
Chapter	1	The Cerebral Cortex	2
Chapter	2	Extrapyramidal System	10
Chapter	3	Posterior Cranial Fossa	14
Chapter	4	Blood Supply of the Brain	21
Chapter	5	Spinal Cord	30
Chapter	6	Peripheral Nervous System	37
Chapter	7	Basis for Localization of Lesions	47
Chapter	8	Lesions of the cerebral Cortex	53
Chapter	9	Lesions of the basal ganglia	82
Chapter	10	Lesions of the posterior fossa	97

Chapter 11 Lesions of the Spinal Cord	111
Chapter 12 Lesions of the Peripheral Nervous System	122
Chapter 13 Lesions of the Neuromuscular Junction and Muscles	136
Chapter 14 Mapping and Identifying Pathology	143
Chapter 15 Laboratory Investigations	155
Chapter 16 Radiologic Investigations	173
Chapter 17 Electro Diagnostic Investigations	206
Chapter 18 Tissue Diagnosis	221
Chapter 19 Guide to Investigation	226

PART 1

BRIEF ANATOMY OF THE NERVOUS SYSTEM

CHAPTER 1

THE CEREBRAL CORTEX

1.0 INTRODUCTION

The nervous system comprises two main parts. These are the central nervous system and the peripheral nervous system. The central nervous system is made up of the brain and spinal cord. The peripheral nervous system is the nervous system outside the brain and the
spinal cord.

1.10 The Cerebrum

The cerebrum is the most developed aspect of the brain in man. It is made up of; the cerebral cortex, the basal ganglia, and their connections. The cerebrum basically is made up of two hemispheres which are slightly joined in the midline. The medial longitudinal fissure divides the two hemispheres.

One hemisphere is slightly larger than the other and is referred to as *the **dominant hemisphere.*** This dominant hemisphere is the left hemisphere in more than 95% of right handed persons and in 60 % of those who are left handed. Each hemisphere is made up of of grey matter, white matter, blood vessels for example the Circle of Willis, cerebrospinal fluid (C.S.F.) and other CSF filled spaces. However, the grey and white matters are the main nervous structures of the cerebrum.

White Matter of Cerebral Hemispheres

The white matter is made up of nerve fibres. These are located within each cerebral hemisphere, underneath to the cerebral cortex. Primarily, the white matter connects the cerebral cortex with other brain regions and identical areas in the two hemispheres. The white matter therefore acts like the connective tissue of the brain. White matter lesions (e.g. Multiple sclerosis) cut across many structures in the central nervous system.

There are three categories of white matter as follows:

The projection fibres originate from the white matter to terminate in other white or grey matter.
The association fibres are fibres that interconnect different regions of the cerebral cortex within one hemisphere.
The commissural fibres interconnect identical areas in the two hemispheres (pleural of cortex). The largest bundle of these commissural fibres is the corpus callosum.

Grey Matter of Cerebral Hemispheres
The grey matter is composed of neurons and forms the largest portion of the brain's total mass. It includes the cerebral cortex, thalamus, hypothalamus, as well as the basal ganglia.

1.20 The Cerebral Cortex
The cerebral cortex is the largest grey matter and forms the most superficial layer of the cerebral hemisphere. It is divided on topographical and functional grounds into four lobes.

These are as follows;

The Frontal lobe
The Parietal Lobe
The Temporal lobe
The Occipital lobe

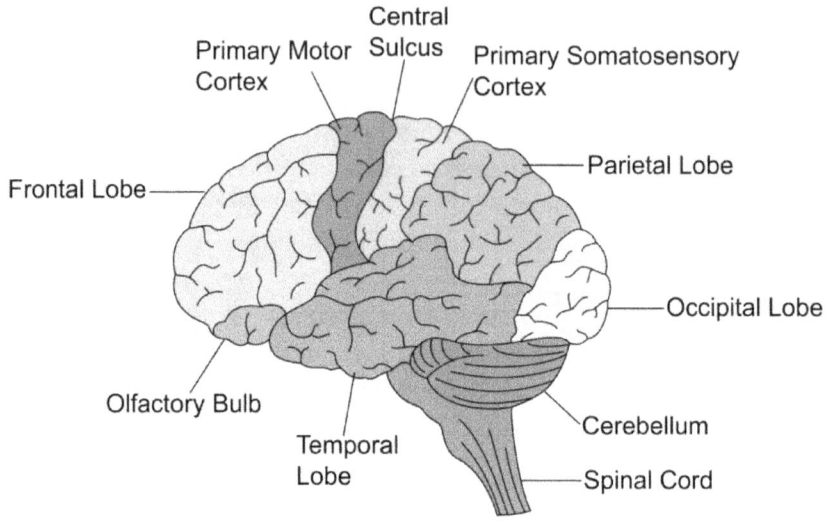

Fig 1 The Brain
(Culled from *https://www.dreamstime.com/stock-illustration-parts-brain-labelled-illustration-image82709486*)

1.21 The Frontal lobe

The frontal lobe is the largest lobe in the brain and includes all the cortex anterior to the central sulcus of Rolando. It is separated from the parietal lobe by the **central sulcus**, and from the temporal lobe by the **lateral sulcus**.The frontal lobe is generally where higher executive functions including emotional regulation, planning, reasoning and problem solving occur. This is why personality changes are often the earliest signs in frontotemporal dementia.Traditional classification systems divide the frontal lobes into the following important areas :

The motor cortex

The primary motor area is the precentral cortex (the strip immediately anterior to the central or Sylvian fissure). It occupies a large part of the precentral gyrus and produces isolated movements on the opposite side of the body. The somatotopic representation in the motor cortex shows an inverted and disproportionate to the size of the lips, tongue, face, and hands on the lower lateral surface. This explains why versive seizures involve the arm, face, with associated tonic eye and neck deviation. It is also explains the greater affectation of the arm more than the leg in cases of anterior cerebral artery infarcts.

The premotor cortex
The premotor cortex lies anterior to the precentral gyrus and the adjoining lower part of the frontal gyri. The functions of the premotor cortex are diverse and not fully understood.

Frontal Eye field
The frontal eye field (FEF) is a region located in the frontal cortex: anterior to the premotor cortex. It controls conjugate movement of the eyes as well as voluntary eye movements. The FEF communicates with extraocular muscles indirectly via the paramedian pontine reticular formation. *Unilateral destruction of the FEF causes deviation of the eyes to the ipsilateral side.*

Broca's speech area
The Broca's area is located around the posterior part of the inferior frontal gyrus of the dominant (usually the left) hemisphere. It is commonly associated with the production of speech (expression). In the damage of the Broca's area, there is difficulty in expression. Such persons are unable to express themselves though they are typically able to comprehend words and sentences. Speech production is sparse with associated word-finding hence they are not fluent. *Stuttering has also been associated with under activity in Broca's area.*

Frontal association cortex (the prefrontal cortex)
The prefrontal cortex extends from the frontal poles to the precentral cortex and includes the frontal operculum. This is made up of a considerable part of the frontal lobe and is one of the remarkable developments of the human brain.

Components of the prefrontal cortex include: orbitofrontal cortex, ventrolateral prefrontal cortex, dorsolateral prefrontal cortex, medial prefrontal cortex (containing the anterior cingulate gyrus, and prelimbic and infralimbic cortices), and the caudal prefrontal cortex (which includes the frontal eye fields). Each of these areas has widespread connectivity. The prefrontal cortex therefore integrates complex perceptual information from sensory and motor cortices. It has a role in maintaining an individual's "personality." The afflicted individual often has difficulty carrying out complex behaviours that are appropriate to the circumstances. The resultant effect is perceived as a change in the patient's "character."

1.22 The Parietal Lobe/ Sensory Cortex
The parietal lobe lies behind the frontal lobe, separated by the central sulcus. The name comes from the Latin word *(paries)* which means "wall". Three anatomical boundaries define the parietal lobe as follows:
The first is the *central sulcus* which separates the parietal lobe from the frontal lobe.
The second is the *parieto-occipital sulcus* which separates the parietal and occipital lobes.
The third and last is the *lateral sulcus (Sylvian fissure)* which is the most lateral boundary and separates the parietal lobe from the temporal lobe. Areas in the parietal lobe are responsible for integrating sensory information, including touch, temperature, pressure and pain. The important cortical areas of the parietal lobe are as follows:

The primary somato-sensory cortex

The post central gyrus which is also called the primary somatosensory cortical area lies immediately posterior to the central sulcus. It is the most anterior part of the parietal lobe. It receives afferent fibres from the thalamus and is concerned *with all forms of somatic sensation*. The postcentral sulcus separates this area from the posterior parietal cortex. The posterior parietal cortex can be subdivided into the superior parietal lobule and the inferior parietal lobule.

The superior and inferior parietal lobules are the primary areas of body or spatial awareness. Therefore a lesion commonly in the right superior or inferior parietal lobule leads to hemineglect.

The parietal association cortex, comprising the remainder of the parietal lobe, is concerned largely with the recognition of somatic sensory stimulation and their integration with other forms of sensory information.

1.23 The Temporal lobe

The temporal lobe is located beneath the Sylvian fissure on both cerebral hemispheres of the mammalian brain. It is separated from the occipital lobe by a line drawn vertically downwards from the upper end of the *lateral sulcus*. The temporal lobe is involved in processing sensory input into derived meanings for the appropriate retention of visual memory, language comprehension, and emotion association. The following are the important areas of the lobe:

The auditory cortex. The fibres of this cortex are from the medial geniculate body. It is concerned with the perception of auditory stimuli.

The temporal association cortex. The temporal association cortex is the part surrounding the auditory cortex and is responsible for the recognition of auditory stimuli and integration with other sensory modalities.

The parahippocampal gyrus

The parahippocampal gyrus is the most medial part of the under surface of the temporal lobe. Most of it is referred to as the entorhinal cortex (EC). It is related anteriorly to the olfactory cortex and is in direct continuity with the *hippocampus* which occupies the whole length of the floor of the inferior horn of the lateral ventricle and extends to the amygdala.

The parahippocampal gyrus is the main interface between the hippocampus and neocortex. The EC-hippocampus system plays an important role in declarative memory. It is particularly important in spatial memories viz formation, consolidation, and optimization in sleep. *Bilateral hippocampal damage results in inability to form new memories.* This is the part of the temporal lobe that is damaged in Alzheimer's disease.

Amygdala

The amygdaloid nuclear complex is also a prominent temporal lobe structure, situated immediately rostral to the hippocampus. Destruction of the amygdala is particularly associated with reduced aggressive behaviour. In addition, the very high density of benzodiazepine receptors in the amygdala also suggests an involvement of the amygdala in anxiety, stress and their treatments.

1.24 The Occipital lobe

The name derives from the overlying occipital bone, which is named from the Latin *ob* behind, and *caput*, the head. It lies behind the parietal and temporal lobes. The Y-shaped *calcarine* and *postcalcarine sulci* are found on the medial aspect. The occipital lobe is the visual processing center. It therefore contains most of the anatomical region of the visual cortex (Striate cortex). There are regions outside the striate cortex (extra striate cortex) that are specialized for different visual tasks, such as visuospatial processing, colour differentiation, and motion perception. Bilateral lesions of the occipital lobe can lead to cortical blindness (Anton syndrome). The following areas of the occipital cortex are noteworthy:

The **visual cortex** surrounds the calcarine and postcalcarine sulci and receives its afferent fibres from the lateral geniculate body of the thalamus of the same side; it is concerned with vision of the opposite half of the visual field.

The **occipital association cortex** lies anteriorly to the visual cortex. This area is particularly concerned with the recognition and integration of visual stimuli.

References

1. Harold Ellis: Clinical Anatomy 11th Ed Oxford 2006
2. https://en.wikipedia.org/wiki/Cerebral_cortex
3. https://www.quora.com
4. Kasper DL, Fauci A S, Hauser S L, Longo D L, Jameson J L, Loscalzo J: Harrison's Principles of Internal Medicine; 19th Ed New York 2015
5. Lindsay K W. Bone I: Neurology and Neurosurgery Illustrated 4th Ed Edinburgh 2005
6. Rohkhamm R. Colour Atlas of Neurology 2ND Ed Stuttgart 2004
7. University of Texas: Neuroscience online, an electronic textbook for NeuroSciences

CHAPTER 2

THE EXTRAPYRAMIDAL MOTOR SYSTEM

2.0 Introduction

This motor system is called extrapyramidal (outside the pyramids). This helps to differentiate it from the tracts of the motor cortex which pass through the medullary pyramids. By definition it should include all those motor projections which do not pass physically through the medullary pyramids. However, the cerebellum is not considered part of the extrapyramidal system despite its involvement in the precision of movements. The most important extrapyramidal structures are the basal ganglia which are involved in complex aspects of motor control; including motor planning and the initiation of movement. Basal ganglia pathologies are therefore associated with a variety of disorders in movement. Hence they are generally called *movement disorders*.

The extrapyramidal tracts actually include tracts that transverse the brain stem to the spine *(bulbospinal tracts)* as follows:
Rubrospinal tract (From the red nucleus)
Reticulospinal tracts (From the reticular formation)
Lateral vestibulospinal tract (From the vestibular tract)
Tectospinal tract (From the tectum)

2.10 The Basal Ganglia (Basal nuclei)

These are structures located in the forebrain. They have associations with the cerebral cortex, thalamus, brainstem and other parts of the brain. They control of voluntary muscle movements. They are also involved in everyday behaviours and habits as well as procedural memory. These habits include the grinding of the teeth, eye movements, cognition and emotion.

The following structures make up the basal ganglia:
Caudate nucleus
Putamen
Globus pallidus
Claustrum

The caudate nucleus and the putamen comprise the striatum. The putamen and the globus pallidus on the other hand make up the lentiform (lens like) nucleus.

Two other structures have similar functions with the basal ganglia: substantia nigra and subthalamic nucleus. *However they are not part of the basal ganglia structurally*. The substantia nigra is actually a component of the brain stem. The subthalamic nucleus on the other hand is closely related to the thalamus.

2.20 The Diencephalon

The diencephalon which is also called the *inter brain* is located between the cerebral hemispheres and brain stem; surrounding the 3rd ventricle. It is the link between the nervous system and the endocrine system and is made up of the hypothalamus and thalamus.

2.22 The hypothalamus

The hypothalamus (*under*, thalamus) is below the thalamus and forms the floor of the third ventricle. It contains a number of small nuclei with a variety of functions. One such function is connecting the nervous system to the endocrine system through the pituitary gland. The hypothalamus is also a part of the limbic system. It is responsible for the regulation of certain metabolic processes and other activities of the autonomic nervous system. The hypothalamus controls body temperature, hunger, and parenting and attachment behaviours. It also controls thirst, fatigue, sleep and circadian rhythms.

2.23 The pituitary gland (hypophysis cerebri)

The pituitary gland is below the hypothalamus in the cavity of the pituitary fossa. It is a protrusion from under the hypothalamus at the base of the brain. The gland rests on the sphenoid bone in the middle of the middle cranial fossa. It is surrounded by a small bony cavity referred to as the sella turcica. The dural fold (diaphragma sellae) covers the gland. The optic chiasma is above the pituitary fossa.

The pituitary is an organ that has two diverse parts ('two in one') organ. The anterior lobe (adenohypophysis) is larger and originates from Rathke's pouch. It regulates many processes. Some of them are stress, growth, reproduction, and lactation. There is an intermediate lobe which synthesizes and secretes melanocyte-stimulating hormone. The posterior pituitary (or neurohypophysis) on the other hand is smaller. It is connected to the hypothalamus through the pituitary stalk. The pituitary stalk is also called the infundibular stalk or the infundibulum. *The posterior pituitary does not produce any hormone.* However it stores and releases two hormones produced by the hypothalamus: Oxytocin and Antidiuretic hormone. Pathologies of the pituitary gland cause many endocrine disorders. Occasionally a tumour grows from remnants of the epithelium of the Rathke's pouch (craniopharyngioma). These tumours are often cystic and calcified.

2.24 The thalamus

Thalamus actually means *chamber*. It is a small mass of grey matter. It is found on top of the brain stem and actually forms the lateral wall of the third ventricle. It is a midline symmetrical structure. The thalamus is the principal sensory relay nucleus which projects impulses from the main sensory pathways onto the cerebral cortex.

References

1. Harold Ellis: Clinical Anatomy 11th Ed Oxford 2006
2. https://en.wikipedia.org/wiki/Basal_ganglia
3. Rohkhamm R. Colour Atlas of Neurology 2ND Ed Stuttgart 2004
4. University of Texas: Neuroscience online, an electronic textbook for NeuroSciences

CHAPTER 3

THE POSTERIOR CRANIAL FOSSA

3.0 INTRODUCTION

There are two structures in the posterior fossa. These are
The Brainstem
The Cerebellum

3.10 The Brain Stem

This structure is actually like a stalk (a stem as the name implies). It forms a link between the cerebral cortex to the spinal cord. In fact, the brain stem is continues as the spinal cord.
It is made up of
The Midbrain,
The Pons
The Medulla Oblongata

These three structures are closely related to the cerebellum. Some authorities include the diencephalon as part of the brain stem.
The corticospinal (pyramidal) tract, the posterior column-medial lemniscus pathway, spinocerebellar and the spinothalamic tract all pass through the brain stem. In essence, the brain stem is like a conduit for all the tracts. The brainstem is also a vital structure for basic survival because it contains essential vasomotor centres: important in the regulation of cardiac and respiratory functions. It also gives rise to the majority of the cranial nerves (ten pairs). In addition the brain stem also contains the reticular formation which plays a pivotal role in maintaining consciousness and regulating the sleep cycle.

3.11 The Midbrain
The midbrain is small and is actually the shortest member of structures in the brain stem It is only 25mm in length which is less than 1 inch. The midbrain connects the pons and cerebellum to the diencephalon. It is divided into three parts: tectum, tegmentum, and the ventral tegmentum. The tectum (*roof*) forms the ceiling of

the midbrain. There are four small structures on the surface of the brain stem. These are referred to as the corpora quadrigemini. There are two superior colliculi and two inferior colliculi. *The upper two(superior colliculi) are involved with vision.* The tectospinal and tectobulbar tracts arise from these superior colliculi. These tracts are responsible for the movements of the neck, head and eye. These movements are important in ability to turn the eyes and necks suddenly and unexpectedly. The two inferior colliculi are smaller. They are associated with audition.

The cerebral peduncles are the only parts of the midbrain actually seen from the front. The substantia nigra which functions as part of the basal ganglia is located deeply in these cerebral peduncles. The substantia nigra also contains the red nucleus. The red nucleus has a connection with the spine (the rubrospinal tract). This rubrospinal tract is *an accessory motor pathway. It acts in controlling arm swing as well as crawling in babies.* The occulomotor and trochlear nuclei are also found in the midbrain.

The tegmentum is the lower part of the midbrain. It contains some nuclei, tracts, as well as the reticular formation. The paired cerebral peduncles are also in the tegmentum.

The Pineal Gland
The pineal gland secretes melatonin. It is not part of the brain stem. However, it is discussed here because it is flanked by the two superior colliculi. It is attached to the thalamus. It secretes melatonin. Melatonin is very important in ensuring the circadian rhythm.

3.12 Pons
The pons is the middle structure of the brain stem. It is in between the medulla oblongata and the midbrain. The pons is recognized as an obvious round structure on the anterior aspect of the brain stem. All the tracts that travel from the cerebral cortex through the medulla to the cerebellum pass through the pons. Sensory signals travelling to the thalamus also pass through the pons. The cerebellar peduncles connect the pons to the cerebellum. The pons also contains the pontine respiratory group. This is made up of respiratory pneumotaxic center and apneustic center.

Basilar portion

The anterior two thirds of the pons is referred to as the basilar pons. One of its functions is to transmit bundles of the corticospinal tract which comes down from the primary motor strip of the cerebral cortex. These fibres are carried to the spinal cord accompanied by corticonuclear fibres. They are called the descending tract. The abducens, facial and vestibulocochlear nerves emerge from the basilar pons at the pontine medulla junction. The trigeminal nerve however emerges at the level of the mid pons.

Pontine Tegmentum (dorsal pons)

The posterior part of the pons is also known as the tegmentum like in the midbrain. It contains the pontine reticular formation alongside several cranial nerve nuclei and ascending spinal tracts. The **loci coerulei** are also located in the rostral pons. The loci coerulei are the main site for the synthesis of noradrenaline in the brain. They also form part of the reticular activating system.

3.13 The Medulla oblongata

The medulla oblongata is generally referred to as the medulla. It is continuous with the pons superiorly and the spinal cord inferiorly. The medulla like the pons also contains the cardiac, respiratory, vomiting and vasomotor centres dealing with heart rate, breathing and blood pressure. These are collectively referred to as the vital centers. The respiratory centre is particularly vulnerable to compression, injury or poliomyelitis with consequent respiratory failure. The medulla has an anterior median fissure in the middle while the medullary pyramids lie laterally. These pyramids contain the fibers of the corticospinal tract. The decussation of these fibres mark the transition from the medulla to the spinal cord is in between the medullary pyramids. Other structures in the medulla are the hypoglossal, glossopharyngeal, vagus and accessory nerve rootlets and the olives. The olives are swellings in the medulla that contain various nuclei and afferent fibers.

The posterior median sulcus contains the innermost part of the medulla. The fasciculus gracilis, and the fasciculus cuneatus are lateral to the posterior median sulcus. The gracile and cuneate tubercles are above these fascicules respectively. The obex is above the gracile and cuneate tubercles. Another important structure in the medulla is the facial colliculus which contains motor nucleus of the facial nerve. These fibres also circle over the nucleus of the abducens (CN VI).The vertebral arteries directly supply the medulla. In addition the medulla is also supplied the posterior inferior cerebellar artery (PIC). This is a branch of the vertebral artery. Infarct of the PICA causes a characteristic syndrome known as Wallenberg syndrome.

3.14 The Reticular Formation

The reticular formation is scattered all over the brainstem. They are nuclei which are intertwined. There is no clear cut anatomic definition. It stretches from the upper part of the midbrain to the lower part of the medulla.

The reticular formation includes ascending pathways to the cortex in the *ascending reticular activating system (ARAS)* and descending pathways to the spinal cord via the *reticulospinal tracts* of the descending reticular formation. The ascending reticular activating system plays a crucial role in maintaining behavioural arousal and consciousness while descending reticulospinal tracts mediate distinct cognitive and physiological processes.

General functions of the reticular formation

Somatic motor control
The maintenance of tone, balance, and posture especially during body movements is a function of the rectospinal tracts.

Cardiovascular control
The reticular formation includes the cardiac and vasomotor centres of the medulla oblongata.

Pain modulation
The reticular formation is also involved in pain modulation. Pain signals emanate from the lower body and travel to the cerebral

cortex. These signals travel via the reticular formation. Hence pain can be increased or reduced by manipulation of this pathway. This makes it the source of the descending analgesic pathways.

Sleep and consciousness
The reticular activating system has an important function in consciousness. This is because it has reticular formation has twigs to the thalamus and cerebral cortex. Therefore, an injury to the reticular formation can cause loss of consciousness.

Habituation
The brain has a way of ignoring meaningless stimuli which are repetitive. However, it remains sensitive to some other stimuli. This process is referred to as habituation and is a function of the reticular activation system.

3.20 The Cerebellum

The larger part of the posterior fossa is occupied by the cerebellum. The cerebellum therefore is the biggest part of the hind-brain. It is behind the fourth ventricle, the pons and the medulla oblongata. It is separated from the cerebral cortex by the tentorium cerebelli. The cerebellum is divided into two hemispheres. It also contains a narrow midline zone known as the vermis.

Most of the cerebellum is made up of a very tightly folded layer of grey matter: the cerebellar cortex. Each ridge or gyrus in this layer is called a *folium*. The cerebellar white matter has a tree like appearance hence it is called *arbor vitae* (tree of life). Within the white matter are four deep cerebellar nuclei, composed of grey matter. The three cerebellar peduncles connect the cerebellum to different parts of the nervous system as follows: to the midbrain by the superior cerebellar peduncles, to the pons by the middle cerebellar peduncles and to the medulla by the inferior cerebellar peduncles.
Functionally, the cerebellum is divided into three parts. These are

Archicerebellum (vestibulocerebellum)

The archicerebellum is also called the vestibulocerebellum. This is because it is closely intertwined in function with the vestibular nuclei. It is made up of the flocculus, nodulus referred to as floccunodular lobe together) and a part of the vermis. The main function of the archicerebrum is the maintenance of equilibrium as well as the coordination of eye, head, and neck movements. Lesions of the archicerebellum lead to vertigo.

Paleocerebellum (Midline vermis)

The paleocerebellum is the middle aspect of the vermis. It is involved in the coordination of the movements of the trunk and leg. Hence it maintains balance and equilibrium. Lesions in the paleocerebellum Vermis lesions result in abnormalities of stance and gait.

Neocerebellum (Lateral hemispheres)

The neocerebellum is actually the posterior part of the cerebellum. Hence it is also referred to as the posterior lobe. The neocerebellum is involved in voluntary control of motor movements. They are particularly involved the control of the fine coordination and dexterity of the limbs especially the upper limbs.

Features of cerebellar disease occur on the same side of the lesion. The dentate nucleus and superior cerebellar peduncle are of utmost importance in the functions of the cerebellum. In fact, the destruction of any of these two structures causes severe disease. The severity is equivalent to the destruction of the whole cerebellar hemisphere.

The infarct of the posterior inferior cerebellar artery gives rise to a characteristic syndrome called Wallenberg syndrome. The features are ataxia and hypotonia of the ipsilateral limbs due to involvement of the inferior cerebellar peduncle and cortex. There will also be cranial nerve (Trigeminal to Vagus nerve) palsies. In addition, there is contralateral loss of pain and temperature sensations.

3.30 The Membranes of the Brain (The Meninges)

There are three membranes surrounding the spinal cord. These are the dura, arachnoid and pia mater. These membranes continue upwards as coverings to the brain.

The *dura* is a dense membrane which, within the cranium, is made up of two layers and forms four sheets :

The falx cerebri
The falx cerebelli
The tentorium cerebelli
The diaphragma sellae

The *arachnoid* is a delicate membrane separated from the dura by the potential *subdural space*. It projects only into the longitudinal fissure and the stem of the lateral fissure.
The *pia* is closely aligned to the outline of the brain. The subarachnoid is the space between the pia and arachnoid membranes. This space is contains the cerebrospinal fluid.

3.40 The ventricular system and the cerebrospinal fluid circulation

The cerebrospinal fluid (C.S.F.) is a clear colourless fluid that is present in the brain and spinal cord. It is produced by the epithelium which covers the choroid plexuses in the ventricles. It circulates through the ventricular system of the brain. The C.S.F drains into the subarachnoid space from the roof of the 4th ventricle. Eventually the C.S.F is reabsorbed into thevenous system of the dura.
In certain areas the subarachnoid space is enlarged generously. These enlargements form the cisterns. Some of thses cisterns are the *cisterna magna, cisterna pontis.* the *interpeduncular cistern,* the *cisterna ambiens,* the *chiasmatic cistern and the quadrigeminal cistern.*

The C.S.F. has may functions in the nervous system. Cardinal amongst them is protection. The C.S.F forms a water-jacket that provides protection for the brain and spinal cord. The C.S.F also helps to regulate the intracranial pressure based on changes in the cerebral blood flow. In the adult, the total volume of C.S.F is about 150 mls. There is about 25mls of C.S.F. in the theca of the spinal cord.

The C.S.F. therefore is normally under a pressure of about 100 mm of water (with a range of 80–180) in the lateral horizontal position. Obstruction to the system causes increased intracranial pressure and ventricular dilatation (hydrocephalus). The analysis of the C.S.F. is very important in diagnosis.

References
1. Harold Ellis: Clinical Anatomy 11th Ed Oxford 2006
2 https://en.wikipedia.org/wiki/Cerebellum
3. https://en.wikipedia.org/wiki/Reticular_formation
4 .Rohkhamm R. Colour Atlas of Neurology .2ND Ed Stuttgart 2004
6. Swash M, Glynn M: Hutchinson Clinical Methods 22nd Ed Edinburgh 2007
7. University of Texas: Neuroscience online, an electronic textbook for NeuroSciences

CHAPTER 4

BLOOD SUPPLY OF THE BRAIN

The proportion of the weight of the brain to that of the whole body is only 2 %. However, as much as 15-20% of the total cardiac output goes to the brain. In essence, the brain is a highly vascularized organ. This explains the severe destructive consequence of cerebrovascular disease. There are two major arteries that supply the brain. These are the common carotid arteries and the subclavian arteries.

4.10 The common carotid arteries
The blood supply of head and neck comes from the common carotid arteries. The two arteries do not originate from the same site. The origin of the *left common carotid artery* is the aortic arch. On the other hand, the origin of the *right common carotid artery is* at the bifurcation of the brachiocephalic artery. After this slight difference, both arteries are similar till they terminate.

Both arteries climb in the carotid fascia in the neck. The carotid sheath also contains the internal jugular vein and the vagus nerve. The cervical sympathetic runs behind the carotid fascia. These four structures are closely related. The common carotid arteries do not give off side branches. Their terminal branches are the external and internal carotid arteries. In size, the two arteries are equal. This termination occurs at the fourth cervical vertebral level (C4).

4.11 The internal carotid artery
The major artery to the brain is the internal carotid artery. It is one of the terminal branches of the common carotid. Its dilatation at this point forms the carotid sinus. This artery maintains the close relationship with the internal jugular vein, vagus nerve and cervical sympathetic chain found in the neck. *The internal carotid artery does not give off any branches in the neck.* However, it gives off some branches on entering the skull. The *ophthalmic artery is a very important branch.* It is the first branch and originates immediately after the carotid sinus. It gives blood supply to the orbital contents. It also gives supply to the skin over the eyebrow.

The most important branch of the ophthalmic artery is the *central artery of the retina*. It is the only blood supply to the retina.

The internal carotid artery has two terminal branches. These are the *anterior* and *middle cerebral arteries*.
The *anterior cerebral artery* gives supply to the medial and superolateral aspect of the cerebral hemisphere.
The *middle cerebral artery* enters the lateral cerebral sulcus, gives off central branches to supply the internal capsule. It also gives supply to most of the lateral aspect of the cerebral cortex and is commonly referred to as 'the *artery of cerebral haemorrhage*'.

4.20 The subclavian arteries
The subclavian arteries do not have similar origins. The *left subclavian artery* takes it origin from the arch of the aorta. The *right subclavian artery* on the other hand is formed by the bifurcation of the brachiocephalic artery. Both subclavian arteries however run a similar course thereafter and give off three main arteries: the vertebral artery, thyrocervical trunk and the internal thoracic artery.

4.21 The vertebral artery
This is the most important of the branch of the subclavian artery. The two vertebral arteries join in front of the pons to form the *basilar artery*.
The following are the important branches of the vertebral artery:
The Anterior and posterior spinal arteries
The Posterior inferior cerebellar artery

The branches from the Basilar Artery are as follows:
The Anterior inferior cerebellar artery
The Superior cerebellar artery
The Posterior cerebral artery

In addition, in the neck, the vertebral artery gives off spinal branches to the cervical spinal cord and vertebrae and muscular branches.

4.22 Circle of Willis

The circle of Willis is a union of different arteries from the cerebral circulation. The internal carotid (anterior circulation) and the vertebra-basilar (posterior circulation) systems meet in the circle of Willis. This circle of Willis ensures some collateral circulation in the brain. In essence, in the event of stenosis or blockage of any artery, there is compensation from the circle. This helps to preserve perfusion of the brain to some extent.

The following are parts of the circle:

The two anterior cerebral arteries (ACA)
The anterior communicating Artery (ACoA)
The two internal Carotid arteries (ICA)
The two posterior cerebral arteries (PCA)
The two posterior communicating arteries (PCoA)
N/B
The middle cerebral arteries are not components of the circle.

The circle of Willis is rarely ever complete. However, it is fully present in some individuals. The circle of Willis is formed at the bifurcation of the internal carotid arteries. The anterior communicating artery (ACoA) forms the link between the two anterior cerebral arteries (ACA). The two posterior cerebral arteries (PCA) arising from the basilar artery form the posterior aspect of the circle. The posterior communicating arteries (PCoA) link the PCAs to the anterior circulation. One PCoA links the PCA to the middle cerebral artery while the other links the PCA to the internal carotid artery. It is common to have variations to this basic structure.

Summary of the blood supply of the brain

In view of the frequent involvement of the pyramidal tract in cerebrovascular accidents, its blood supply is listed here in some detail:

Motor cortex
leg area: anterior cerebral artery
face and arm areas: middle cerebral artery
Internal capsule: branches of the middle cerebral artery;

Cerebral peduncle: posterior cerebral artery;
Pons: pontine branches of basilar artery;
Medulla: anterior spinal branches of vertebral artery;
Spinal cord: segmental branches of anterior and posterior spinal arteries.

4.30 Veins and venous sinuses of the brain

The cerebral venous system
Two different systems ensure the venous drainage of the brain. The first is the dural sinus which drains the superficial structures. The cerebrum and cerebellum drain into adjacent sinuses.
The internal cerebral veins however drain the deep structures. Two main veins unite to form the internal cerebral vein. The first is the choroid vein. The choroid plexus is drained by the choroid vein as the name implies. The second is the thalamostriate vein. The basal ganglia drain into this vein. The great cerebral vein (vein of Galen) is a merger of the two internal cerebral veins. The great cerebral vein merges with the inferior sagittal sinus to form the straight sinus.

4.31 The venous sinuses of the dura
The venous sinuses lie between the layers of the dura. They receive the venous drainage of the brain and of the skull (the *diploic veins*) and empty into the internal jugular vein. They also communicate with the veins of the scalp, face and neck via *emissary veins*.
The venous sinuses are as follows:

The *superior sagittal sinus* lies along the attached edge of the falx cerebri and ends posteriorly in the right transverse sinus.

The inferior sagittal sinus lies in the free margin of the falx cerebri and opens into the straight sinus.
The *straight sinus* lies in the tentorium cerebelli along the attachment of the falx cerebri.

The transverse sinuses commence at the internal occipital protuberance and run in the tentorium cerebelli on either side. The transverse sinuses become the sigmoid sinuses and eventually emerge from the jugular foramen as the internal jugular vein.

The cavernous sinuses
The cavernous sinuses are very important in clinical practice. They are found on the body of the sphenoid on both sides. However, the two cavities freely communicate through the intercavernous sinuses. The carvenous sinus has very close relations with the carotid artery as well as certain cranial nerves. These are Occulomotor, Trochlear, Abducens and the Ophthalmic and maxillary divisions of Trigeminal. Other closely related structures are the optic tract, the uncus of the temporal lobe and the internal carotid artery. These structures are on top of the cavernous sinus. The sinus drains the ophthalmic, superficial middle cerebral, sphenoparietal and the petrosal veins. The cavernous sinus is susceptible to sepsis and thrombosis which leads to severe cavernous sinus thrombosis disease.

4.32 The internal jugular vein
The internal jugular vein is actually an extension of the sigmoid sinus. It originates at the jugular foramen and ends behind the clavicle. It forms the brachiocephalic vein together with the subclavian vein. It is related to the internal carotid at first and subsequently the common carotid artery in the carotid fascia.

The following veins are tributaries of the internal jugular vein: the pharyngeal venous plexus, the common facial vein, the lingual vein and the superior and middle thyroid veins.

Superficial veins
The head and neck have many superficial veins. These are organised in diverse ways. All of them drain to either the external or internal jugular veins. The majority of them unite to form the external jugular vein. The rest of the veins unite to form the facial vein. The facial vein is one of the tributaries of the internal jugular vein.

4.40 Blood Brain Barrier
The blood brain barrier (BBB) is a highly selective semi permeable membrane. It separates the circulating blood from the brain

and extracellular fluid in the central nervous system (CNS). It occurs along all capillaries and is made up of tight junctions around the capillaries that do not exist in normal circulation. The blood–brain barrier (BBB) is formed by the brain capillary endothelium. Despite similarities with the blood cerebrospinal fluid barrier and the blood retinal barrier (BRB), the BBB is extremely different. The blood–cerebrospinal fluid barrier is a function of the choroidal cells of the choroid plexus. On the other hand, the blood–retinal barrier specifically protects the retina. It is destroyed by Diabetes retinopathy.

Circumventricular organs
There are certain structures in the brain that are not covered by the BBB. These are called the circumventricular organs. The sensory circumventricular organs are the area postrema (AP), the subfornical organ (SFO) and the vascular organ of lamina terminalis. The secretory organs include the sub commissural organ (SCO), some parts of the pituitary gland, the median eminence, and the pineal gland. The secretion of melatonin is "directly into the systemic circulation".
Other structures outside the BBB include the roof of the third and fourth ventricles. These structures are therefore not 'protected' by the BBB.

Functions
The function of the BBB is the prevention of neurotoxins into the brain. These are usually lipophillic. However it allows the passage of water, some gases, and lipid-soluble molecules, glucose and amino acids that are crucial to neural function.
Hence, it protects the brain from most pathogens. The few exceptions are *toxoplasma gondii*, *Borrelia*, Group B streptococci and *Treponema pallidum*.
Blood-borne infections of the brain therefore are very rare but are often serious and difficult to treat when they occur. The BBB also prevents approximately 100% of large-molecule neuro therapeutics and more than 98% of all small-molecule drugs from entry into the brain. It also prevents antibodies which are too large to cross the blood–brain barrier.

The BBB however becomes more permeable during inflammation thereby allowing some antibiotics and phagocytes to move across the BBB. Hence it is difficult to treat brain diseases once the BBB is functioning. Many mechanisms have been tried. These include going either "through" or "behind" the BBB, use of endogenous transport systems (glucose, amino acids carriers) and the use of Mannitol. Currently the new technology (Nanotechnology) is in consideration. In addition the use of peptides may also be helpful.

4.50 Lymphatic drainage

It is a long standing belief that the human brain has no lymphatic drainage system. Recent findings show that functional lymphatic drainage does exist in the brain. It is composed of basement membrane-based perivascular pathway, a brain-wide lymphatic pathway, and cerebrospinal fluid (C.S.F.) drainage routes including sinus-associated meningeal lymphatic vessels and olfactory/cervical lymphatic routes. The brain lymphatic system serves as a route of drainage for interstitial fluid (ISF) from brain parenchyma to nearby lymph nodes. It also helps to maintain water and ion balance of the ISF, waste clearance, and reabsorption of macromolecular solutes. It is thought that the impairment and dysfunction of the brain lymphatic system has crucial roles in age-related changes of brain function. Other effects are in the pathogenesis of neurovascular, neurodegenerative, and neuro inflammatory diseases, as well as brain injury and tumors.

References

1. Harold Ellis: Clinical Anatomy 11th Ed Oxford 2010
2. https://www.ncbi.nlm.nih.gov/pubmed/28903061
3. https://www.sciencedirect.com/science/article/pii/S0301008217300 62
4. Kasper DL, Fauci A S, Hauser S L, Longo D L, Jameson J L, Loscalzo J: Harrison's Principles of Internal Medicine; 19th Ed New York 2015 Illustrated 4th Ed Edinburgh 2005
5. Rohkhamm R. Colour Atlas of Neurology 2ND Ed Stuttgart 2004
6. Ropper AH, Brown R H: Adams and Victor' Principles of Neurology 8th Ed New York 2005
7. University of Texas: Neuroscience online, an electronic textbook for NeuroSciences

CHAPTER 5

THE SPINAL CORD

5.0 Introduction

5.10 The Spinal Cord

The second part of the central nervous system is the spinal cord. It is located within the spine. It is a bundle of nerves which is long and thin measuring 18in (45cm) long. The cord begins superiorly at the foramen magnum in the skull, where it is continuous with the medulla oblongata of the brain and terminates in the lumbar region. There are thirty one pairs of spinal nerves. These are attached along the entire length of the spinal cord. There is a disparity between the length of the spinal cord and the spine. This makes the length of the roots to increase progressively downwards.

The spinal cord takes up the whole length of the spinal canal in utero. This is so till the third month of fetal life. It is after this that the vertebral bones start growing faster than the cord. The tip of the spinal cord corresponds to the third lumbar vertebra at the time of birth. With further growth, the difference between the length of the cord and spine increases gradually. In an adult, the cord is between the first and second lumbar vertebrae. Below the second lumbar vertebrae, the nerve roots form the *cauda equina* (tail of the horse). This is shown in the diagram in Fig 2.

The spinal cord like the brain is also protected by the meninges. The outermost layer is called the dura. It is very tough. The stability of the cord is a function of the dura. This is done through the denticulate ligaments. The space between the dura and the bone is full of adipose tissue and a network of blood. It is called the epidural space. The next and middle layer is the arachnoid. It has a mesh-like appearance. The pia mater is the innermost and final layer. It is very delicate and lines the surface of the spinal cord. The subarachnoid space is the space between the pia and arachnoid. It contains the cerebrospinal fluid (C.S.F.)

5.11 The Conus Medullaris

The terminal tip of the spinal cord is called the conus medullaris (Latin for "medullary cone"). Rarely, it is also called the conus terminalis (terminal cone). It is located in within the first and second lumbar vertebral bones. Occasionally it may be lower. The upper borders however are not well defined. It is characteristically tapered.

Filum terminale

A prolongation of the pia mater known as the filum terminale (internum) arises from the apex of the conus medullaris and gets attached to the back of the coccyx. The filum terminale thereby provides a connection between the conus medullaris and the coccyx which stabilizes the entire spinal cord.

5.12 The Cauda Equina

The lower spinal nerves form a tail referred to as the cauda equina (from Latin *horse's tail*). It includes nerve pairs from the second lumbar, all the sacral and the coccygeal nerve. The nerve fibres gradually decline in number as individual pairs leave the spinal column. These nerves innervate the pelvic organs and lower limbs and the sphincters. It also innervates of perineum and partially parasympathetic innervation of the bladder.

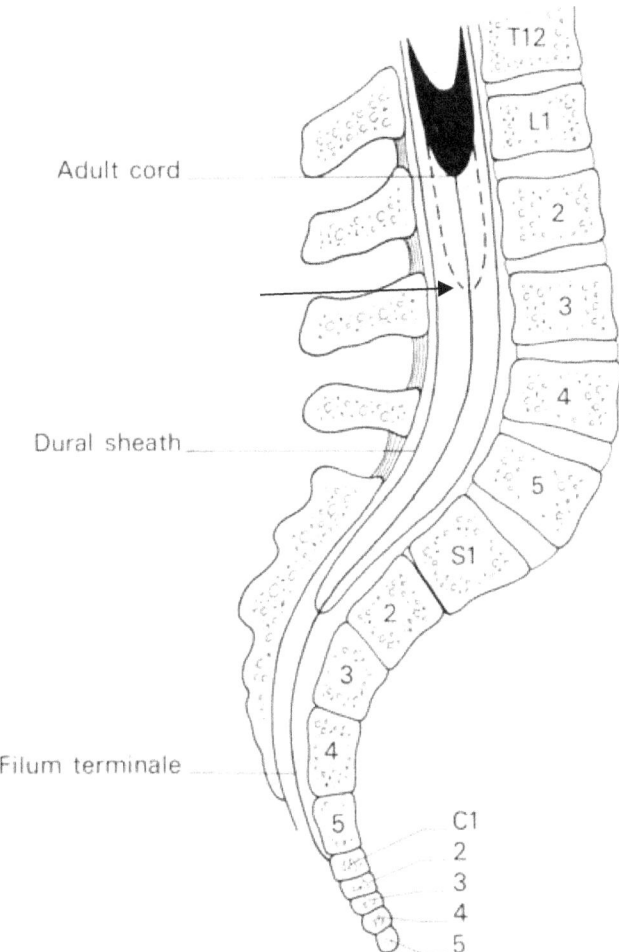

Fig 2 The Spinal cord in adulthood

(Culled from Clinical Anatomy 13th Ed by Harold Ellis)

5.20 The Descending tracts

The pyramidal (lateral cerebrospinal or crossed motor or corticospinal tract) tract.

The pyramidal is the main 'voluntary' motor pathway and at such the most popular of all the tracts. It is made up of the corticospinal and some corticobulbar tracts. Most of the pyramidal tracts are derived from the motor area of the cerebral cortex. However the rest(one thirds) arise from the somatosensory cortex. It originates from the pyramidal cells of the motor cortex. This explains the name: pyramidal tracts. The tract runs through the subcortical white matter (internal capsule) through the brain stem and decussates in the medulla (about 70-90% of the fibres). It finally descends on the contralateral side of the cord.The pyramidal tract therefore is the only crossed motor tract. At *each spinal segment*, fibres enter the anterior horn ; where there is a synapse. The tract therefore becomes progressively smaller as it descends. After the synapse the fibres continue to the innervated muscle. Note that there is no synapse before the anterior horn cells. Hence the fibres from the motor cortex to the anterior horn cells before the synapse are referred to as upper motor neurones(also called first order neurones) while the fibres after the synapse are referred to as the lower motor neurones (second order neurones).

The direct pyramidal (anterior cerebrospinal or uncrossed motor) This is a small tract (the remaining 10-30%) descending without medullary decussation. At each segment, however, fibres pass from this tract s to the ventral horn (anterior) motor cells of the opposite side.

5.30 The Ascending tracts
The ascending tracts start from the body and climb up to the brain.

The ascending tracts are as follows:
Posterior and Anterior Cerebellar Tracts
The Lateral and Anterior Spinothalamic Tracts
The Posterior Columns

The posterior and *anterior spinocerebellar tracts*
The spinocerebellar tracts originate from the spine as the name implies. They ascend on the same side of the cord and enter the cerebellum through the inferior and superior cerebellar peduncles respectively.

The lateral and *anterior spinothalamic tracts*
The lateral and anterior tracts carry the pain and temperature sensory modalities. These fibres enter the spinal cord through the the posterior roots. Thereafter, they ascend for a few segments. Subsequently, the fibres cross over to the opposite side to ascend to the thalamus. They eventually get relayed at the sensory cortex.

The posterior columns
The posterior columns form the medial fasciculus gracilis (of Goll) and a lateral fasciculus cuneatus (of Burdach). At the medulla, they decussate and synapse. The fibres pass to the thalamus and finally relay in the sensory cortex. The posterior columns convey sensory fibres that subserve fine touch and proprioception (joint position sense) and vibration.

5.40 Blood supply to the Spinal Cord

Vertebral arteries
The vertebral arteries are the main source of blood to the spinal cord. However, the following arteries branch from the vertebral arteries to directly supply the spinal cord itself:
One anterior spinal artery
Two posterior spinal arteries
Anterior and posterior radicular arteries
Arterial vasocorona (anastomose between the spinal arteries)
The *single* anterior and two posterior spinal arteries are direct branches of the two vertebral arteries. They merge to form the basilar artery. Thus, the vertebral arteries are very important, as they serve as the primary source of blood to the brain and the spinal cord.

References

1. Epstein RJ. Medicine for examinations 4th Ed Canada 2006
2. Harold Ellis: Clinical Anatomy 11th Ed Oxford 2006
3. https://en.wikipedia.org/wiki/Spinal_cord
4. Rohkhamm R. Colour Atlas of Neurology 2ND Ed Stuttgart 2004
5. Ropper AH, Brown R H: Adams and Victor' Principles of Neurology 8th Ed New York 2005
6. Swash M, Glynn M: Hutchinson Clinical Methods 22nd Ed Edinburgh 2007
7. University of Texas: Neuroscience online, an electronic textbook for NeuroSciences

CHAPTER 6

THE PERIPHERAL NERVOUS SYSTEM (PNS)

6.0 Introduction

The second part of the nervous system is known as the peripheral nervous system (PNS). The PNS is composed of nerves and ganglia which are neither part of the brain nor the spinal cord. The PNS links the central nervous system with the other structures in the body. The PNS is not covered or protected by the skull, spine or the BBB. Hence it is vulnerable to injuries from many sources. This includes mechanical injuries, chemicals and toxins.

6.10 Structure of the Peripheral nervous system

The peripheral nervous system has two components:
The somatic nervous system
The autonomic nervous system

6.20 The Somatic Nervous system

The somatic nervous system is the voluntary limb of the PNS. This is because, it can be controlled voluntarily. The function of this system is the transmission of signals from the brain to end organs. The somatic nervous system is made up of afferent (sensory) nerves and efferent (motor nerves). Many of the nerves however perform both functions. The cranial nerves carry all information (both sensory and motor) in the head and neck.

There are twelve cranial nerves. Ten of these originate from the brainstem. These cranial nerves control the functions of the anatomic structures of the head. However, there are some exceptions. The 31 spinal nerves control the functions of the rest of the body.

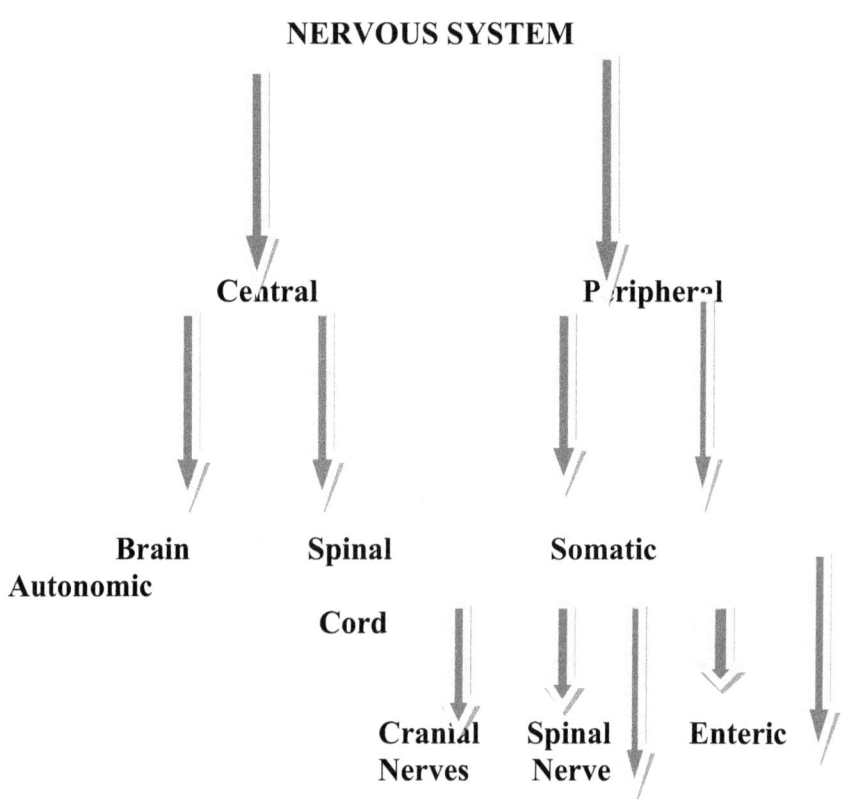

Fig 3: Organization of the nervous system

The Cranial Nerves

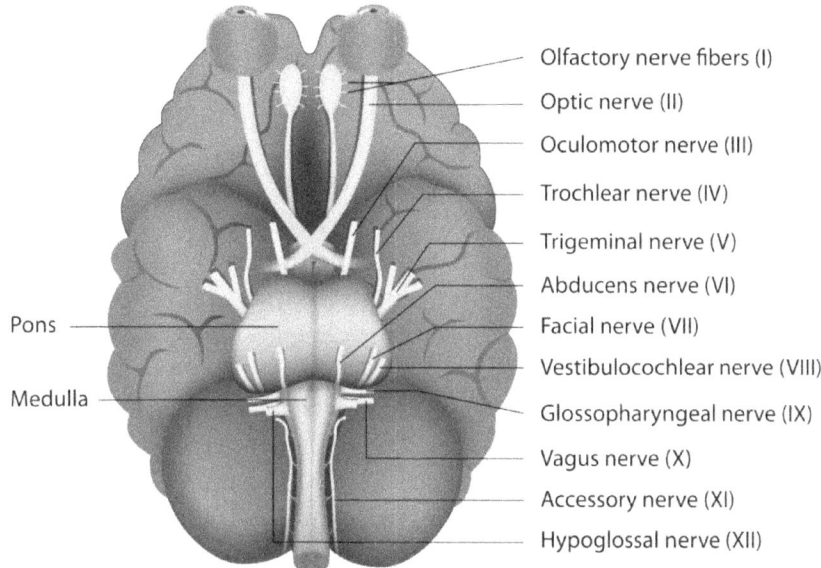

Fig 4 The roots of the cranial nerves
(Culled from https://www.dreamstime.com/stock-images-12-cranial-nerves-image24625974)

6.30 THE CRANIAL NERVES

6.31 The Olfactory nerve (I)

The olfactory nerve has a distinct characteristic. The fibres are actually the central of cells. They are not peripheral processes from the ganglion. These central processes move up through the cribiform plate of the ethmoid bone. They synapse in the olfactory bulb. These axons eventually relay in the cortex. In humans, the sense of smell is not well developed. This means that it can be distorted with relative ease. Hence conditions affecting the nasal mucosa generally (e.g. the common cold) disturb the sense of smell. However, unilateral anosmia is an important sign in the diagnosis of frontal lobe tumours.

6.32 The Optic nerve (II) and the visual pathway

The optic nerve is the nerve of vision. It is actually not a true cranial nerve but rather a brain tract drawn out from the cerebrum. The optic nerve passes to the optic foramen and reaches the optic groove on the dorsum of the body of the sphenoid. At the optic chiasma, there is a decussation. All the fibres from the inner half of the retina cross over. The fibres at the outer half continue on the same side. The crossed over fibres are responsible for the vision in the temporal (outer) field. The fibres that did not cross over are responsible for the vision in the nasal (inner) field.

This cross over at the optic chiasma explains the unique visual loss in lesions that compress the optic chiasma. Most of the fibres in the optic tract end up in the six-layered *lateral geniculate body* of the thalamus. A small proportion which subserves pupillary, ocular and head and neck reflexes, bypasses the geniculate body to reach the superior colliculus and pretectal area. From the lateral geniculate body the fibres move to the temporal lobe before passing backwards to the occipital visual cortex.

6.33 The Occulomotor nerve (III)

The occulomotor nerve is very important in the control of eye movements. It supplies most of the extrinsic eye muscles and the preganglionic parasympathetic fibres for the sphincter of the pupil via the ciliary ganglion. The nerve originates from the cerebral aqueduct. This occurs at the level of the superior colliculus. The occulomotor nucleus is made up of two components.

These are the *somatic efferent nucleus*, which supplies the ocular muscles and the *Edinger–Westphal nucleus* from which the preganglionic parasympathetic fibres are derived.

6.34 The Trochlear nerve (IV)

The trochlear nerve is also the fourth cranial nerve and the only cranial nerve to originate from the posterior aspect of the brainstem. This nerve which is also the thinnest of all the cranial nerves supplies only one muscle. This is the *superior oblique* muscle. Diplopia occurs when there is weakness of the superior oblique muscle as a result of trochlear nerve injury. This happens when the person looks sideways and down. It is referred to as 'the tramp's nerve" because it makes the eye go "down and out"!

6.35 The Trigeminal nerve (V)

The trigeminal nerve is also the fifth nerve. As the name implies, is made up of three divisions. Most of the sensation to the head and face are supplied by the branches of the fifth nerve. They also supply the mucous membranes of the mouth, nose and paranasal air sinuses and the muscles of mastication. Four autonomic ganglia, the ciliary, pterygopalatine, otic and submandibular are associated with this nerve.
.
Branches of the Trigeminal Nerve
V1: The ophthalmic division
This is the smallest division of the trigeminal nerve; it is wholly sensory and is responsible for the innervation of the skin of the forehead, the upper eyelid, cornea and most of the nose.
V2: The maxillary nerve
The maxillary nerve is also a purely sensory nerve like the ophthalmic.
V3: The mandibular nerve
This is the largest of the three nerves. It is also the only one to convey motor fibres. There are structures that receive sensory supply from the mandibular nerve. These include the temples, lower face, anterior two thirds of the tongue and the floor of the mouth. The muscles of mastication receives motor supply. It also supply the salivary glands(secretomotor).

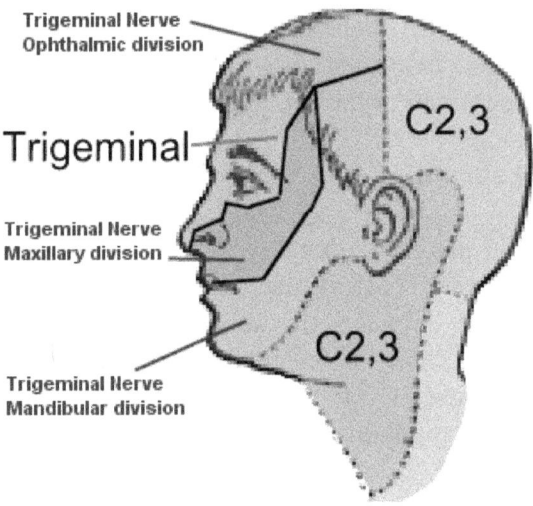

Fig 5 The supply of the Trigeminal branches
(Culled wellnessadvocate.com)

The Nuclei of the 5th nerve

The fifth nerve has both sensory and motor nuclei. The sensory nuclei are very big and are the *largest of the cranial nerve nuclei.*
They are found in the entirety of the brain stem as well as the cervical cord. The nuclei comprise three parts. Each one is involved with a different sensory modality.
The parts are
The Chief sensory nucleus
The Descending or spinal
The Mesencephalic nucleus

The chief sensory nucleus has many other names. These are "pontine nucleus", "main sensory nucleus", "primary nucleus" or "principal nucleus". This nucleus is concerned with touch. The spinal trigeminal nucleus is in charge of pain and temperature. The mesencephalic nucleus is involved with proprioception. The separate trigeminal motor nucleus is medial to the chief sensory nucleus.

6.36 The Abducens nerve (VI)

The abducens nerve like the trochlear nerve also supplies only one eye muscle. This is the *lateral rectus*. Its nucleus is in the lower aspect of the pons. The main characteristic of the nerve is a long nerve convoluted course in the brain. This makes it a target for raised intracranial pressure and basal skull injuries.

6.37 The facial nerve (VII)

The facial nerve which is the seventh supplies the muscles of facial expression. It also supplies salivary and lacrimal glands (secretomotor fibres). It also supplies the nasal mucosa. In addition, it carries taste fibres from the anterior two-thirds of the tongue. The facial and abducens nerves form the facial colliculus. They also have a relationship with the vestibulocochlear nerve in the cerebellopontine angle. The sensory and motor fibres pass together into the internal auditory meatus and enter the facial canal. Prior to the synapse at the nucleus, the corticofacial fibres give a bilateral innervation to the lower part of the face. These are the upper motor neurones. The upper part of the face on the other hand is mainly innervated by the neurones after the synapse. These are the lower motor neurones. This is the basis for distinguishing upper and lower motor neurone lesions of the facial nerve which is pertinent in the localization of the lesion.

6.38 The Auditory (Vestibulocochlear) nerve (VIII)

The 8th nerve has two sets of fibres: cochlear and vestibular. The *cochlear fibres* are concerned with hearing. Most of the efferent fibres ascend in the lateral lemniscus to the *inferior colliculus* and the *medial geniculate body*. All the fibres eventually relay on *the auditory cortex*.

The *vestibular fibres* (concerned with equilibrium) enter the medulla and terminate in the *vestibular nuclei*. Many of the efferent pass to the cerebellum. Other vestibular connections are to the nuclei of III, IV, VI and XI and to the upper cervical cord (via the vestibulospinal tract). These connections bring the eye and neck muscles under reflex vestibular control.

6.39 The Glossopharyngeal nerve (IX)
The glossopharyngeal nerve gives sensory supply for the pharynx and the posterior one-third of the tongue. This includes including the taste buds, stylopharyngeus muscle and parotid gland. Another branch called the carotid nerve supplies both the carotid body and carotid sinus.

6.40 The Vagus nerve (X)
The vagus nerve has the widest distribution of all the cranial nerves. It innervates the heart and the major part of the respiratory and alimentary tracts. The fibres that supply the muscles of the soft plate, pharynx and larynx are from the nucleus ambiguus. Hence the examination of the palatal muscles remains a good test for the integrity of the Vagus nerve. In unilateral paralysis, the uvula deviates to the normal side when the patient says 'Ah'.

6.41 The Accessory nerve (XI)
The accessory nerve has two separate roots; cranial and spinal. This nerve innervates the sternocleidomastoid as well as the trapezius muscles.

6.42 The Hypoglossal Nerve (XII)
The hypoglossal nucleus is found in the fourth ventricle. The nerve which has only motor functions exits the brainstem from the medulla. Almost all the muscles of the tongue receive their supply from the hypoglossal nerve. The only exception is the palatoglossus muscle. There is an ipsilateral paralysis in the event of injuries of the hypoglossal nerve. In addition, there is associated wasting of the muscles of the tongue.

6.50 The Spinal Nerves

6.51 Introduction
All nerves that originate from the spinal cord instead of the brain) are referred to as spinal nerves. The result from a web ("plexus") interrelated nerves roots which get organized to form single nerves. The spinal nerves control the functions of the whole body apart from the face, neck and some parts of the head. A total of thirty one (31) pairs of nerves make up the spinal nerves in human

beings. The components of the spinal nerves include eight cervical nerves, twelve thoracic nerves and five lumbar nerves. In addition, there are also five sacral nerves and one coccygeal nerve. These nerves are named according to the adjacent spinal vertebrae. The nerve roots cervical section exit above corresponding vertebrae. However, the nerve roots exit below the corresponding vertebrae from the thoracic to the coccygeal sections.

The total number of the cervical vertebrae is seven. The nerve that originates between C7 and T1 is called referred to spinal nerve root C8. The spinal nerve roots in the lumbar and sacral sections are within the dural sac. They form a bundle beneath the second lumbar vertebrae. This looks like a tail and is aptly called the cauda equina (tail of the horse).

6.52 Cervical spinal nerves (C1–C4)

The four cervical nerves make up the cervical plexus. This plexus is inside the sternocleidomastoid muscle in the neck. The plexus generates many nerves that supply the back of head and neck. These include the superior occipital nerve, the greater and lesser occipital nerves along with the greater and lesser auricular nerves. The nerve roots of the third to fifth cervical vertebrae generate the phrenic nerve. The phrenic nerve supplies the thoracic diaphragm, enabling breathing. Spontaneous breathing is impossible if the spinal cord is transected above the third cervical vertebrae (C3).

6.53 Brachial plexus (C5–T1)

The nerves arising from the last four cervical vertebrae nerves, C5 to C8, and the first thoracic spinal nerve, T1, combine to form the brachial plexus, or plexus brachialis. The brachial plexus is a tangled array of nerves which forms the nerves that subserve the upper-limb and upper back. It is a highly organized network of fibres.

6.54 Lumbosacral plexus (L1–Cocc1)

The anterior divisions of the lumbar nerves, sacral nerves, and coccygeal nerve form the lumbosacral plexus. The first lumbar nerve is frequently joined by the subcoastal nerve which is the twelfth thoracic.

This plexus is divided into three major parts:
Lumbar plexus; supplies the skin as well as muscles of the lower limbs
Sacral plexus; supplies the skin as well as muscles of the pelvis
Pudendal plexus; innervates the external genitalia as well as perineum.

6.60 The Autonomic Nervous System (ANS)

The Autonomic Nervous System is the second part of the peripheral nervous system. It was formerly called the *visceral nervous system*. It is an involuntary system controlled by the hypothalamus which acts as an integrator and it receives input from the limbic system. The medulla is the origin of the autonomic nerves. Autonomic functions are as follows; control of respiration, cardiac regulation and vasomotor activity. Others are reflex actions such as sneezing, coughing, vomiting and swallowing.
The autonomic nervous system has three branches:
The Sympathetic nervous system
The Parasympathetic nervous system
The Enteric nervous system

Every organ in the body has both a sympathetic and parasympathetic supply. Each system generates the opposite effect to the other.

6.61 The Sympathetic Nervous System
The sympathetic nervous system is that empowers the body for emergency situations. Hence it sets up a reaction system by the body which is generally referred to as the "fight or flight" response. Its operations are carried out through a series of interconnected neurons which lie within the central nervous system.
There are two types of sympathetic neurons: Pre-ganglionic and Post-ganglionic.
Pre-ganglionic
These are the neurons before the synapse at the ganglion.
Post-ganglionic
These are the neurons after the synapse at the ganglion.

The pre-ganglionic neurons originate from the first thoracic section all the way to the second or third lumbar segments of the spinal cord. They are generally shorter. They are therefore referred to as having a "thoraco-lumbar outflow". The postganglionic neurons begin after the synapse in the ganglion and spread to the whole body. Activation of the pre-ganglionic neurons leads to a release of acetylcholine which binds and activates nicotinic acetylcholine receptors on the ganglion. In response, postganglionic neurons release noradrenaline (norepinephrine). In some cases, there may be release of adrenaline from the adrenal medulla due to prolonged activation. These catecholamines bind to the adrenergic receptors on peripheral tissues triggering off the fight-or-flight response. This includes pupil dilation, increased sweating, increased heart rate, and increased blood pressure. There is a concomitant reduction in activities which are not critical for survival like digestion.

6.62 The Parasympathetic system

The parasympathetic system activates what is termed the *'rest and digest response'* or *feed and breed*. The action is complementary to the sympathetic nervous system. Nerve fibres of the parasympathetic nervous system arise from specific nerves and include several cranial nerves: the occulomotor nerve, facial nerve, glossopharyngeal nerve, and vagus nerve (3, 7, 9 and 10). Three spinal nerves in the sacrum (S2-4), referred to as the pelvic splanchnic nerves, also act as parasympathetic nerves. It is therefore called the *"craniosacral outflow"*. The parasympathetic system primarily uses acetylcholine as the mediator. It is responsible for stimulation of the activities that occur when the body is at rest, especially after eating, including sexual arousal, salivation, lacrimation (tears), urination, digestion and defecation. Consequently, when the parasympathetic system dominates the body, there is an increase in salivation and activities in digestion, while heart rate and other sympathetic response decrease. *The parasympathetic system has some voluntary control.* This voluntary control is classically seen in control of both urination and defecation. *The sympathetic system on the other hand has no voluntary control.* Notably, these two systems are not dependent on each other. In many cases, both systems have "opposite" actions where one system activates a physiological response and the other inhibits it. This is the reason certain parts of the body can be activated, while others are rested.

Studies in recent times have recognized a third subsystem of neurons. This third system is referred to as non-noradrenergic, non-cholinergic transmitters. Nitric oxide is a neurotransmitter. The system is essential in autonomic function especially in the gut and the lungs.

6.63 The Enteric Nervous System

This is the lesser known division of the autonomic nervous system. It is located only around the digestive tract. The enteric nervous system allows for local control without input from the sympathetic or the parasympathetic branches. The enteric system acts specifically to regulate functions of the gastrointestinal system. The enteric nervous system (ENS) is considered a separate entity from the autonomic nervous system in recent times. This is because it has an independent reflex activity.

References

1. Harold Ellis: Clinical Anatomy 11th Ed Oxford 2006
2. https://en.wikipedia.org/wiki/Sympathetic_nervous_system
3. https://en.wikipedia.org/wiki/Parasympathetic_nervous_systm
4. Kasper DL, Fauci A S, Hauser S L, Longo D L, Jameson J L, Loscalzo J: Harrison's Principles of Internal Medicine; 19th Ed New York 2015
5. Rohkhamm R. Colour Atlas of Neurology 2ND Ed Stuttgart 2004
6. Ropper AH, Brown R H: Adams and Victor' Principles of Neurology 8th Ed New York 2005
7. Swash M, Glynn M: Hutchinson Clinical Methods 22nd Ed Edinburgh 2007
8. Walker HK, Hall WD, Hurst JW; Clinical Methods, the History, Physical, and Laboratory Examinations 3rd Ed Boston 1990
9. University of Texas: Neuroscience online, an electronic textbook for NeuroSciences

PART 2

LOCALIZATION OF LESIONS OF THE NERVOUS SYSTEM

CHAPTER 7

BASIS FOR LOCALIZATION OF LESIONS

7.10 Introduction

The concept of localization of lesions of the central nervous system sounds daunting to medical students and young doctors. This same localization however is done with ease in other systems. The principle of localization is the same irrespective of the system that is involved. Localization simply means *"where is the lesion"* responsible for a patient's symptoms and signs. This anatomical localization precedes the formulation of differential diagnosis and further relevant investigations to confirm the eventual diagnosis. Consequently, ordering an oesophagoscopy or barium meal for a patient with clinical features of right upper quadrant abdominal pains, jaundice and hepatomegaly will be considered outrageous by most medical doctors. This is because the constellation of features is in keeping with not just a gastrointestinal tract disorder but specifically a hepato-biliary disease. It therefore stands to order that the hepato-biliary tract should be the appropriate aspect of the gastrointestinal system to be investigated. Investigating the oesophagus therefore is superfluous, irrelevant and an unnecessary waste of funds. In the same manner, in the central nervous system, a different constellation of symptoms suggests the affectation of a different part of the nervous system. Localization of the lesion therefore requires a good understanding of the anatomy of the nervous system, its blood supply, and the disease processes involved.

Invariably the process of localization should begin during history taking, and refined during the general and neurological examinations. This stepwise process is extremely important as it ensures a narrower spectrum of the possible differentials in the diagnosis. Further information from the biodata (gender, age, race), associated features, past medical, family and social history will assist in defining the possible etiology. Thereafter *relevant* diagnostic studies are carried out for the eventual diagnosis. *No degree of sophisticated neuroimaging, electrophysiologic or laboratory studies and technology should replace the clinician's anatomical localization based on history taking and examination.* The practice of overreliance on investigations is a common pit fall seen in diagnosis in neurological cases.

In fact, it is not uncommon for newly referred patients to present to the neurology clinic clutching a cranial CT scan or an MRI; most of which were irrelevant in the first place or inappropriate. A person with a myopathic gait may walk in with an MRI scan of the brain: the myopathic gait indicates proximal myopathy so why scan the healthy brain? Another common mistake is to order the correct neuroimaging study but the wrong site or protocol. Commonly, a lumbo- sacral MRI for patients is mistakenly requested for a patient with paraplegia. The adult spinal cord ends at the first lumbar vertebra as shown in chapter 5. In essence, there is no spinal cord in the lumbar and sacral segments, thus the lumbar sacral segment is the wrong site to investigate when the clinical features suggest a spinal cord lesion. The appropriate investigation will be an MRI of the thoracic spine if there is paraparesis/paraplegia. In cases of quadriparesis /quadriplegia then the cervical is the appropriate segment to be investigated.

In addition, lesions may go undetected on standard imaging studies hence, the studies should be specifically focused on the anatomical location involved. In some cases, neuroimaging or laboratory studies may disclose incidental abnormalities that have no bearing on the patient's symptoms and the further pursuit of which can lead to unnecessary time, expense, and potentially patient harm. This is unethical considering the fact that most of these neuroimaging studies are expensive and unavailable in many instances especially in poor resource settings.

Furthermore a good number of neurological disorders do not need investigations to confirm diagnosis e.g. Parkinson disease, Trigeminal Neuralgia, primary headaches, Tetanus, Rabies Encephalitis. In order to identify the anatomic location, a good knowledge of the anatomy of the nervous system is imperative. *Attention to the patient's description of symptoms usually helps in the accurate localization of the lesion.* A more detailed examination of a particular region of the CNS or PNS is often indicated after taking the history. **Note that a second examination is the best tool in a difficult neurological case.**

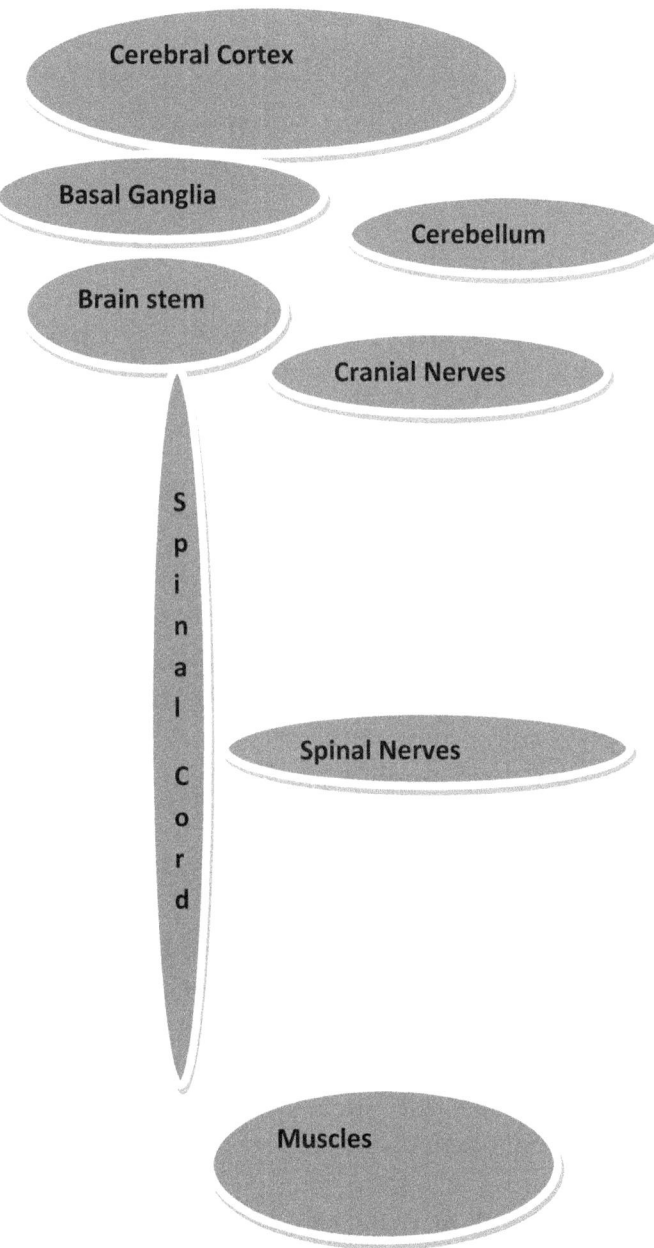

Fig 6 Divisions of the neuraxis

7.10 Steps in the localization of CNS Lesions are;

1. What is/are the site(s) of the lesion(s)?
2. Mapping out the lesion
3. What is the likely pathology/aetiology?
4. What is the clinical diagnosis?

7.20 Define the Anatomy

The first step in localization is to define which part of the nervous system is involved. The divisions of the neuraxis are shown in Fig. 6. All the diseases of the nervous system will involve at least one of the structures in the neuraxis. It is pertinent to define whether the lesion is in the central nervous system (CNS), the peripheral nervous system (PNS), or both? If in the CNS, is the pathology in the cerebral cortex, sub-cortical white matter, basal ganglia, brainstem, cerebellum, or spinal cord?

Are the pain-sensitive meninges involved? If in the PNS, could the disorder be located in peripheral nerves and, if so, are motor or sensory nerves primarily affected, or is the lesion in the neuromuscular junction or muscle?

7.30 Mapping out the Lesion
In mapping out the lesion, the symptoms and the temporal profile are extremely important. These will help to define whether the lesion, focal, multi focal or diverse?

7.40 What is the pathology and aetiology?
Further history of associated features, past medical history, family and social history will give a clearer view of the pathologic process involved and possible aetiology of the disease.

7.50 Make a clinical diagnostic formulation
In view of the foregoing, the clinician makes a diagnostic formulation and possible differential diagnosis.

References

1. Biller J, Grener G, Brazis PW. De Meyer's the Neurologic Examination: A programmed Text 7th Edition.www.neurology.mhmedical.com Mc Graw –Hill Education
2. Ekeh Bertha C; Clinical Neurology made Easy 1st Ed USA 2018
3. http://www.human-memory.net/types_declarative.html
4. Howlett Neurology in Africa Bergen, Norway 2012
5. Kasper DL, Fauci A S, Hauser S L, Longo D L, Jameson J L, Loscalzo J: Harrison's Principles of Internal Medicine; 19th Ed New York 2015
6. Lindsay K W. Bone I: Neurology and Neurosurgery Illustrated 4th Ed Edinburgh 2005
7. Ropper AH, Brown R H: Adams and Victor' Principles of Neurology 8th Ed New York 2005
8. Swash M, Glynn M: Hutchinson Clinical Methods 22nd Ed Edinburgh 2007
9. Zazulia A R. Neurological Diagnosis & Localization; https://neuro.wustl.edu/education/medical-student-education/neurology-clerkship/localization/

CHAPTER 8

LESIONS OF THE CEREBERAL CORTEX

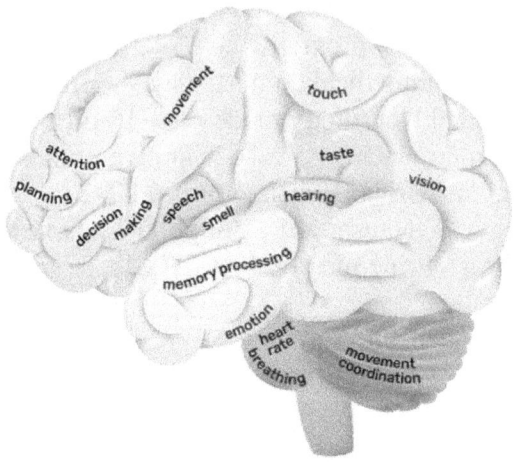

Fig 7 The cerebral cortex
(Culled from https://qbi.uq.edu.au/brain/brain-anatomy/lobes-brain)

8.0 Introduction
There are four main lobes in the cerebral cortex;;
The Frontal lobe
The Parietal lobe
The Temporal lobe
The Occipital lobe

These lobes have their different functions as shown in fig 7 above. Therefore, looking at the diagram above, one can briefly draw the inference as follows;

1. Lesions of the frontal lobe will affect movement, speech, attention, planning and decision making.
2. Lesions of the parietal cortex will affect sensation and taste.
3. Lesions of the temporal lobe will affect smell, hearing, memory processing and emotions.
4. Lesions of the occipital lobe will affect vision.

The reality however is more complex than the above simple summary. This is because though the cerebral cortex contains approximately 20 billion neurons spread over an area of 2.5 m2, *the primary sensory and motor areas constitute only 10% of the cerebral cortex*. The remaining 90% is occupied by the association cortex which *is made up of the* cerebral cortex *outside the primary areas. In essence, the association cortex is much larger than the corresponding primary cortex. The association areas are also by far the most developed part of the cerebral cortex and the brain in general.*
Furthermore, the association cortex is essential for mental functions that are much more complex. The association cortex therefore mediates the integrative processes that subserve cognition, emotion, and comportment. Current concepts have shown that there are no specific centres for "hearing words," "perceiving space," or "storing memories." Higher cortical functions (domains) are therefore said to *be coordinated by intersecting large-scale neural networks that contain interconnected cortical and subcortical components.*

Five anatomically defined largescale networks are noted to be the most relevant to clinical practice. These are:

(1) Perisylvian network
(2) Parietofrontal network
(3) Occipitotemporal network
(4) Limbic network
(5) Prefrontal network

8.10 The Perisylvian network

The is a network around the Sylvian fissure (perisylvian network) region of the left hemisphere. this is the main site for language. It is made up of the Broca's and Wernicke' areas. The Broca's area located in the inferior frontal gyrus. The Wernicke's area on the other hand is located in the posterior parts of the temporal lobe. Difficulty in fluency, phonology, and the grammatical structure of sentences are noted when there is damage to the Broca's area. Damage to the Wernicke's area interferes with the ability to understand spoken or written sentences as well as the ability to express thoughts through meaningful words and statements. The two language areas are interconnected with each other as well as with surrounding parts of the frontal, parietal, and temporal lobes. Disorders of in the perisylvian area lead to an impairrment in language. this is referred as *dysphasia*. *Aphasia* is the more commonly used terminology. It actually means total destruction of language. this may affect either the production or comprehension of speech as well as the ability to read or write. In view of the fact that the preference of one hand (handednes)is located in the dominant hemisphere usually the left, most people have aphasia after lesions of the left hemisphere. This will incude as much 95% of those who are right handed and 65% of those who are left handed.The unusual case where the aphasia is occurs after a right hemispheric lesion is referred to as *crossed aphasia.*

8.11 Types of Aphasia

Wernicke's Aphasia
In Wernicke's aphasia (also called Sensory, Receptive or Fluent aphasia), there is an impairment in the comprehension of spoken, written words and sentences.The speech comprises long sentences which have no meaning. The person may also add unimportant words or completely veer off the conversation. In some cases, the patient may even create new "words" (neologisms) which have no meaning (jargon aphasia). In fact the patient often gets angry not realizing that his or her language is incomprehensible. In most cases, gestures and pantomime may not improve comprehension but the ability to follow commands aimed at axial musculature may be preserved.

Broca's Aphasia
The Broca's area in the frontal operculum is the center for expression of language. Broca's aphasia is also called motor, expressive or non-fluent aphasia. The patient speaks short, meaningful phrases that are produced with great effort. In normal individuals the average number of words spoken per minute is 100-115 words, however in Broca's aphasia, the speech is sparse (i.e.

the person speaks 10 to 15 words per minute). Moreover, the speech is made up of nouns, transitive verbs, or important adjectives. In addition, the length of the phrase is shorter with the omission of many of the small words (articles, prepositions, conjunctions). The speech is surprisingly meaningful. In severe cases, the output may be reduced to a grunt or single word. (monosyllabic speech like '*Yes* or *No'*). Comprehension of spoken language however remains intact except for sentences that are difficult.

Conduction Aphasia
Conduction aphasia occurs when there is a disconnection between the Wernicke's and Broca's areas. The person speaks fluently and also comprehends speech. However, such a person may have difficulty with repeating words or sentences. The damage typically involves the arcuate fasciculus and the left parietal region. In naming, there is difficulty in distinguishing speech sounds that make words differ e.g. d' and 't' in food and foot. These are called phonemic paraphasias: the words sound alike but have totally different meanings. In addition, spelling is impaired in conduction aphasia as well as reading aloud while comprehension is preserved.

Global Aphasia
The combined dysfunction in both the Broca's and Wernicke's area is referred to as Global aphasia. It is common is cerebrovascular diseases that involve the entire middle cerebral artery distribution in the left hemisphere. The output of speech is nonfluent, and the comprehension of language is severely impaired. *They can neither understand nor express themselves.*

Anomic Aphasia
Anomic aphasia results from a "minimal dysfunction" syndrome of the language network. Articulation, comprehension, and repetition are intact, but there is impairment of naming; hence the person keeps looking for the correct word (word finding). However, the person does not pause while word finding making the language output fluent. Instead, he or she uses many words to describe one word (circumlocutions). One of the author's patients in trying to say my husband said *"He is the man I live with who is the father*

of my children". In some cases, the words are jumbled and the sentences are meaningless (paraphasias). Hence, there is not much information from the speech. There is also difficulty in spelling. *Anomic aphasia is the commonest language disturbance seen in head trauma. It is also very common in metabolic encephalopathy, and Alzheimer's disease.*

8.12 Transcortical Aphasias: Fluent and Nonfluent

The transcortical aphasias comprise different types of aphasia whose origin is *not localised to the perisylvian area*. They are discussed here because of their similarity with the perisylvian aphasias. Lesions like stroke occuring in between the ACA and MCA (anterior watershed area) cause transcortical aphasias. They also occur as a result of lesions that affect the supplementary motor cortex in the territory of the anterior cerebral artery. Clinical features of fluent (posterior) transcortical aphasia are similar to those of Wernicke's aphasia, *but repetition is intact*. The lesion site appears to be the posterior watershed zone).The features of nonfluent (anterior) transcortical aphasia are similar to those of Broca's aphasia, *but repetition is intact and agrammatism is less pronounced.*

Isolation aphasia represents a combination of the two transcortical aphasias.There is severe impairment of comprehension, and no purposeful speech output. However the patient may continually repeat fragments of conversations spoken by others (*echolalia*). This is an indication that the neural mechanisms for repetition are at least partially intact.The site of lesion is the surrounding frontal, parietal, and temporal cortex. Common causes are anoxia, carbon monoxide poisoning, or complete watershed zone infarctions. These are characteristically patchy.

8.13 Pure Word Deafness

Pure word deafness is also called *auditory agnosia*. It is characterized by great difficulty in understanding spoken words. The ability to repeat spoken words is also lost. The language which is native or at least familiar to the person sounds alien. Surprisingly, they can express themselves well in that same language either spoken or written voluntarily. *They also have no difficulty in understanding the language in a written form*. The most common causes are either bilateral or left-sided middle cerebral artery (MCA) strokes affecting the superior temporal gyrus. The lesion interrupts the flow of information from the auditory association cortex to the language network. The involvement of the cingulate cortex leads to the development of akinetic mutism. Such a person is unable to speak and move.

8.14 Dyslexia/ Alexia

Dyslexia (difficulty with words) is a reading disorder that is characterized by difficulty with reading and or understanding despite normal intelligence. It is the visual equivalent of pure word deafness. There is a marked variability in affectation of different individuals. It remarkably affects the following: spelling of words, reading quickly, writing words, pronouncing and understanding what one reads. The inability to make out or understand written words is often devastating. The person is able to communicate verbally (the intellect is normal). The difficulties seen in dyslexia are involuntary. They are first noticed at school as such children may be considered unintelligent by the teachers. *When someone who previously could read loses the ability, it is known as **alexia**. Hence alexia is the acquired form of dyslexia.*

Certain structures have been identified by imaging as the sites of the lesion. These are the inferior frontal gyrus, inferior parietal lobule, and the middle and ventral temporal cortex. These structures in the left hemisphere of are associated with the ability to read. The lesions interrupt the flow of visual input into the language network. The core language network remains unaffected. Patients with this syndrome also may lose the ability to name colours, although they can match colours. This is known as a *colour anomia*.

8.15 Pragmatics and Prosody

Pragmatics refers to aspects of language that communicate attitude, affect, and the figurative aspect. One component of pragmatics is prosody which refers to variations of melodic stress and intonation that influence attitude of verbal messages giving a different meaning to the same sentence. Damage to right hemisphere regions corresponding to Broca's area impairs the ability to introduce meaning-appropriate prosody into spoken language. The speech has correct grammar with accurate word choice. However the statements are uttered in a monotone with little or no facial expressions. Hence, the ability to convey the intended stress and affect is lost. For example consider the following sentences: Dr *Etim is back. Dr Etim is back? Dr Etim is back!* The three sentences are exactly the same four words but convey different meanings. The first sentence is just the statement of a fact, the second shows surprise and the third is emphatic. Hence the voice stress, intonation and facial expression convey a different meaning to each sentence (prosody of speech). When the prosody of speech is lost, all the sentences will sound the same and the different meanings are lost (aprosodia). The stress, intonation and facial expression in the following sentences should not be the same: I love ice cream (*pleasant*), my mother is dead (*sober/sad*) and I will kill that girl (*defiant*). In aprosodia however all will be altered in similar monotones. The lack of defining voice intonations or facial expression gives the mistaken impression of being depressed or indifferent. This expressive aprosodia is a feature of right opercular lesion.

8.16 Subcortical Aphasia
Subcortical structures like striatum and thalamus are also involved in speech. Damage to these structures can also lead to aphasia.

8.17 Gerstmann's Syndrome
This is the combination of *acalculia* (impairment of simple arithmetic), *dysgraphia* (impaired writing), *finger anomia* (an inability to name individual fingers such as the index and thumb), and left-right disorientation (an inability to tell whether a hand, foot, or arm of the patient or examiner is on the right or left side of the body). It is easily confused with anomia hence generalized anomia and aphasia should be excluded before making a diagnosis of this syndrome. Gerstmann's syndrome is associated with damage to the inferior parietal lobule (especially the angular gyrus) in the left hemisphere. It may occur in isolation or acutely.

8.20 The Parietofrontal Network

The parietofrontal network is a large network. It is made up of the cingulate cortex, posterior parietal cortex, frontal eye fields, striatum and thalamus. They are involved in extra personal space, events as well as motor strategies for attention. Damage to this network causes the impairment of distribution of attention within the extrapersonal space, giving rise to hemispatial neglect, simultanagnosia and object finding failures. Other features are impairments in route finding, the ability to avoid obstacles, and the ability to dress.

8.21 Hemispatial Neglect

This is the inability of a person to recognize one side of the body as his body. Persons with hemineglect may fail to dress, shave, or groom the left side of their body. They are known to hit the left side on doors since they are unable to acknowledge that side of the body. They may also fail to eat food placed on the left side of the tray. Such a person leaves an unusually wide margin on the left while writing. On examination in the clinic, you can draw a horizontal line and ask him to divide it into two (line dissection). He will divide the right side such that the line is divided into ¼ on the right and ¾ on the left. He also circles the letters on one side when given a target with many letters (visual target cancellation). Hemineglect is more common, more severe, and longer lasting after damage to the right hemisphere (non dominant hemisphere) than after damage to the left hemisphere. Severe neglect for the right hemispace is rare.

8.22 Extinction

The failure to appreciate simultaneous stimulations from both sides (visual, auditory or tactile); not recognizing the stimulus from the left is referred to as *extinction.* Some persons with neglect may actually deny the existence of hemiparesis and may even deny ownership of the paralyzed limb, a condition known as *anosognosia.* Hemispatial neglect is also *usually associated with large deficits of attention of the non-dominant hemisphere.*

8.23 Balint's Syndrome

The bilateral involvement of the parietofrontal cortex leads to a state of severe spatial disorientation known as Balint's syndrome. It is an uncommon and incompletely understood triad of severe neuropsychological impairments. Features are occulomotor apraxia, optic ataxia and simultanagnosia.

Occulomotor apraxia is difficulty in scanning the environment and fixating on an object. The person is unable to voluntarily guide his eyes in a desired direction without moving the head.

Optic ataxia
The inability to accurately point to a target is referred to as optic ataxia. The patient is unable to touch an object he is looking at because of a disordered coordination of eye and hand movement. It is especially true with the hand opposite the side of the lesion. Optic ataxia is also called misreaching or Dysmetria (difficulty with lengths).

Simultanagnosia is the inability to view all the features simultaneously. The patient with simultanagnosia sees like the 'six blind men of Hindustan who went to *see* the elephant'. Each blind man could only feel a different part of the elephant and perceived the elephant to be a tree, rope or wall having felt the leg, tail or body respectively. The person with simultanagnosia is unable to see all the details at the same time, (simultaneously). He can therefore call a table lamp an ashtray because he is unable to see the whole lamp but can only see the circular base. Simultanagnosia can occur without the other two components of Balint's syndrome. Some patients with simultanagnosia report that objects they are looking at vanished suddenly. This is because of an inability to look back at the original point of gaze.

8.30 The Occipitotemporal Network

Lesions of the occipitotemporal network cause difficulty in recognition of familiar persons or objects (*agnosia*). The operative word here is recognition. Agnosia may be visual, auditory, or tactile.

8.31 Visual agnosia

The inability to recognize visually presented objects despite the *preservation of elementary sensory functions* is known as visual agnosia. It is caused by extensive occipital damage. There are two main forms of visual agnosia; *apperceptive and associative*.

In **visual apperceptive agnosia**, there is poor or no perception of the object. He has difficulty in assembling parts of an image into a whole picture; no recognition. These persons have difficulty in distinguishing shapes, recognizing or copying the different stimuli. They may describe the parts but are unable to use their past experience to recognize person or object.

In **visual associative agnosia**, the person is unable to match the correct visual percept with previously processed sensory data and recognition. Patients can describe visual scenes and classes of objects but still fail to recognize them. He can call a fork 'spoon': in essence, he can make the association that the object (fork) is a piece of cutlery. This poor recognition in visual associative agnosia may take the form of inability to recognize familiar faces (**prosopagnosia**). A patient with *prosopagnosia* cannot recognize familiar faces, including, sometimes, the reflection of his or her own face in the mirror. Characteristically, they have no difficulty with the generic identification of a face as a face or a car as a car, but may not recognize the identity of an individual face or the make of an individual car (perception of the object is intact).

Agnosia may become generalized and extend to the generic identification of common objects, the condition is known as **visual object agnosia**. Other forms of visual agnosia include failure to recognize familiar voices (**phonagnosia**) and colours (**achromatopsia**). In some cases there is difficulty in recognizing motion (**akinetopsia**).

8.32 Dyslexia/Alexia

Dyslexia as already discussed is the difficulty in the recognition of words. It is actually a type of visual agnosia. The acquired form known as alexia is also called *agnostic alexia*. It is not possible to read with pure alexia since the person is unable to recognize or understand words and written language.

8.33 Auditory agnosia/Pure word Deafness

Auditory agnosia and pure word deafness are one and the same. It actually affects two networks; perisylvian and occipitotemporal. It results from affectation of the superior temporal gyrus leading to the interruption the flow of information from the auditory association cortex to the language network as already discussed in aphasia.

8.34 Tactile agnosia (Astereognosis)

The inability to recognize or identify objects by touch alone is known as tactile agnosia. The person may recognize and feel the weight or texture of the object. However he is unable to describe it or comprehend the significance. Some of the forms are astereognosis which is the inability to identify familiar objects (key, comb, purse, and phone) by touch alone. **Autotopagnosia** is a rare form in which the person is unable to orient the parts of his own body.

8.35 Apraxia/Motor agnosia

Apraxia is a peculiar disorder of skilled movement. It is not caused by weakness, akinesia or deafferentation. There are no abnormal tones, postures or movement disorders such as tremors or chorea. In addition, there is no intellectual deterioration, poor comprehension, or uncooperativeness. *In fact, apraxia is a form of a motor agnosia* hence the discussion here. These patients do not have weakness but have lost information about how to perform skilled movements. Apraxia is an extremely important syndrome in behavioural neurology. However it is not well understood. Persons with apraxia are unlikely to perform activities of daily

living well. Some of the common types are caused by lesions in the left hemisphere and is commonly associated with aphasic syndromes, especially Broca's aphasia and conduction aphasia. In view of this, apraxia may also be discussed with the aphasias.
Apraxia is one of the best localizing signs of the mental status examination and, unlike aphasia, also predicts disability in patients with stroke or dementia.

8.36 Types of Apraxia

Ideomotor apraxia
In ideomotor apraxia, there is difficulty in performing a specific motor act ('cough', 'comb your hair') or pantomime the way to use a common tool (a comb, hammer, straw, or toothbrush). These patients fully understand the commands since there is no impairment in language or hearing.

Buccofacial apraxia/Oral apraxia
This is actually a subset of ideomotor apraxia but the deficits are restricted to the movements of the face and mouth. The person cannot perform skilled actions involving the lips, mouth and tongue (blowing out a match, kissing, licking the lips or whistling) despite intact power.

Sympathetic dyspraxia
Patients with lesions of the anterior corpus callosum can display ideomotor apraxia confined to the left side of the body, a sign known as *sympathetic dyspraxia*. A severe form of sympathetic dyspraxia known as the *alien hand* syndrome is characterized by additional features of motor disinhibition on the left hand.

Ideational apraxia
In ideational apraxia, there is a deficit in the performance of a goal-directed sequence. However there is no difficulty in executing the individual components of the sequence. The best example is the sequence of uncapping the pen and writing. It involves uncap the pen, place the cap at the opposite end, turn the pen point towards the writing surface, write, remove the cap and recap. The patient may either write with a capped pen, write with the wrong

end of the pen. It is worthy of note that he recognizes that the pen is used to write. This is unlike in ideomotor apraxia where the person does not recognize the use of a familiar object or tool. Ideational apraxia is commonly seen in persons with acute confusional states and dementias rather than focal lesions associated with aphasic conditions.

Constructional apraxia: There is inability to draw or copy quality pictures, such as interlocking pentagons, or complex figures. This is a part of the Mini Mental State Examination (MMSE)

Dressing Apraxia: In dressing apraxia, there is inability to dress. The person may pass the head over the sleeve or wear the dress on the inverse side.

Gait apraxia
Gait apraxia is the loss of ability to have normal function of the lower limbs such as walking. There is difficulty in initiation of movement. The person appears glued to the ground when attempting to walk. He also has difficulty in stopping the movement. The power however is normal on examination because there is no weakness of the muscles. The pathology originates from the motor association cortex.

Limb-kinetic apraxia
In limb-kinetic aphasia, there is clumsiness in voluntary movements of the extremities e.g. a person affected by limb apraxia may have difficulty waving.

Occulomotor apraxia is difficulty in scanning the environment and fixating on an object. The person is unable to voluntarily guide his eyes in a desired direction without moving the head despite the fact that such a person has full random eye movements. This is also a component of Balint's syndrome as discussed earlier.

Apraxia of speech (AOS)
There is difficulty in the planning and coordination of the movements necessary for speech (e.g. in saying potato, the person may say topato). AOS can independently occur without issues in

areas such as verbal comprehension, reading, comprehension, writing, articulation or prosody. The severe form of acute speech apraxia is called aphemia.

Aphemia presents with severely impaired fluency (often mutism). Patients with aphemia usually have full recovery though there is an intermediate stage of hoarse whispering. *It is noteworthy that writing, reading, and comprehension are intact, and hence aphemia is not a true aphasic syndrome.*

8.40 The Limbic Network

The limbic system is made up many diverse structures in the brain. These are the limbic and paralimbic areas (such as the hippocampus, amygdala, and entorhinal cortex). Others are the anterior and medial nuclei of the thalamus, some parts of the striatum as well as the hypothalamus. Most of this network was called the Papez circuit but now better defined as a network. The limbic system is in charge of coordination of emotion, motivation, autonomic tone, and endocrine function. In addition, it has a *major role in declarative (explicit) memory for recent episodes and experiences*. The other aspect of memory is a function of the prefrontal network of executive function and behaviour. Noteworthy is that patients with amnestic states can acquire new motor or perceptual skills even though they may have no conscious knowledge of the experiences that led to the acquisition of these skills.

Amnesia

Amnesia is a disturbance in memory *(a not* and *mnesis* remembering*)*. It is often confused with dementia. This is because memory impairment is a core symptom of dementia. In amnesia, the only problem is the loss or impairment of memory. In dementia however, there are other cognitive impairments associated with the memory impairment. In other words, memory impairment is a necessary but not sufficient enough to make a diagnosis of dementia. In addition, the memory loss in dementia is progressive unlike amnesia that is not progressive. Moreover the person with amnesia is able to carry out normal activities of daily living unlike in dementia, where there is a marked impairment in activities of daily living.

8.41 Types of Amnesia
There are two main types of amnesia:
Retrograde amnesia and Anterograde amnesia
Retrograde amnesia is the inability to retrieve information that was acquired before the amnestic state. The memory loss can extend back decades, or only a few months. Relatively recent events are more vulnerable to retrograde amnesia than are more remote and more extensively consolidated events However it is usually temporary and can be treated by exposing them to old memories and treatment of underlying cause.

Anterograde amnesia
Anterograde amnesia is the most important component of the amnestic state. The person has an inability to store, retain, and recall 1new knowledge. In the acute stages, there also may be a tendency to fill in memory gaps with inaccurate, fabricated, and often implausible information. This is known as *confabulation*. Confabulation is commonly seen in Wernicke-Korsakoff syndrome and traumatic head injury. In these conditions, there is an interference of the underlying lesion with the frontal network. These two types of amnesia are not mutually exclusive; both can occur simultaneously.

Other types of amnesia based on specific to aetiology
Post-traumatic amnesia
This is caused by a head injury (a fall, a knock on the head, an assault). It is often transient, but may be permanent. It may be either anterograde, retrograde, or the mixed type.

Dissociative amnesia/Psychogenic amnesia results from a psychological cause usually after an unpleasant, stressful or traumatic experience (Repressed). Such memory is stored in long-term memory, but access to it is impaired because of psychological defense mechanisms. The person however still has the ability to learn new information. Later on, there may be some partial or complete recovery of memory.

Dissociative fugue (*formerly* psychogenic fugue) is also known as fugue state. It is caused by unresolved temporary psychological trauma. The person is confused about his identity or totally unaware in some cases. It is common for such a person to travel far away from familiar surroundings and create new identities.

Transient Global Amnesia
In transient global amnesia, there are no clear precipitating factors. It usually resolves in one day. Proposed possible etiologies include blood flow, seizure or an atypical type of a migraine. Other causes of amnesia include Thiamine deficiency, drugs, temporal lobe epilepsy and post hypnotic. Damage to the limbic network does not necessarily destroy memories but interferes with their conscious recall in a coherent form. The individual fragments of information remain preserved despite the limbic lesions and can sustain the non declarative (*implicit or procedural*) memory. This is because procedural memories do not involve the hippocampus at all. They are rather encoded and stored by the cerebellum and putamen, caudate nucleus and the motor cortex: structures involved in motor control. The putamen is the storage site for learned skills such as driving. Instinctive actions like grooming on the other hand are stored in the caudate nucleus. Generally, timing as well as coordination of body skills remains the functions of the cerebellum.

8.50 The Prefrontal Network

The network for executive function and behaviour is found in the frontal lobe. The frontal lobe has four lobes as already described. The motor component is in control of isolated movements in the opposite side of the body. The other three components jointly referred to as the prefrontal cortex their interconnected subcortical structures (head of the caudate and part of thalamus) make up the network that coordinates exceedingly complex aspects of human cognition and behaviour. The prefrontal network therefore plays an important role in behaviours that require multitasking and the integration of thought with emotion. Lesions involving this network are referred to as *frontal lobe syndromes.*

8.51 Frontal abulic syndrome

In the *frontal abulic syndrome*, there is lack of motivation. The patient shows a loss of initiative, creativity, and curiosity. He is emotionally bland, apathetic, and also lacks empathy.

8.52 Frontal disinhibition Syndrome

In the *frontal disinhibition syndrome*, where there is damage to the orbitofrontal cortex, there is lack of response inhibition. This manifests as severe impairments of judgment, insight, foresight, and the inability to mind rules of conduct. There is a remarkable dissociation between intact intellectual function and a total lack of everyday common sense. The person may remove his clothes or urinate in public. He continually displays these inappropriate behaviours without appearing to feel any embarrassment, pain, guilt, or regret. Other features are impulsiveness, puerility, a jocular attitude, sexual disinhibition, and complete lack of concern for others. In fact, the person with frontal lobe disinhibition syndrome is disliked because he is considered a bad and selfish person. They do not get the kind consideration given to persons with Alzheimer's disease who are considerably older from their relatives.

8.53 Memory

Other areas affected in the damage to the frontal lobe include deficits in attention-related functions like *working memory which is the transient online holding and manipulation of information*. In addition, concentration span, the scanning and retrieval of stored information, the inhibition of immediate but inappropriate responses and mental flexibility are also impaired. Digit span; the ability to recite seven digits forwards and five backwards is impaired. There is disruption of the orderly registration and retrieval of new information.

Memory involves three stages

Registration and encoding
The information is registered followed by an encoding. The memory is therefore like a filing system. If it is not in the file, then it cannot be retrieved. Orderly registration and encoding is affected in the lesions of the prefrontal network.

Storage and retention
The storage of memory for conscious retrieval is important in working memory. The prefrontal cortex functions in the transient online holding and manipulation of the information before the storage.

Recall/Retrieval
Conscious recall or retrieval of needed information is domiciled in the limbic system. Damage to the limbic system causes an inability to recall information. Hence it affects declarative memory which requires conscious retrieval (limbic network). Implicit or procedural memory (prefrontal network) is not affected because such memories have become innate and do not require conscious retrieval. Procedural or implicit memory includes all skills acquired. Procedural memory is encoded and stored by the cerebellum, putamen, caudate nucleus and the motor cortex: structures involved in motor control.

8.54 Classification of Memory

Memory has been classified in many different ways.
Most classify according to duration

Classification of Memory according to Duration

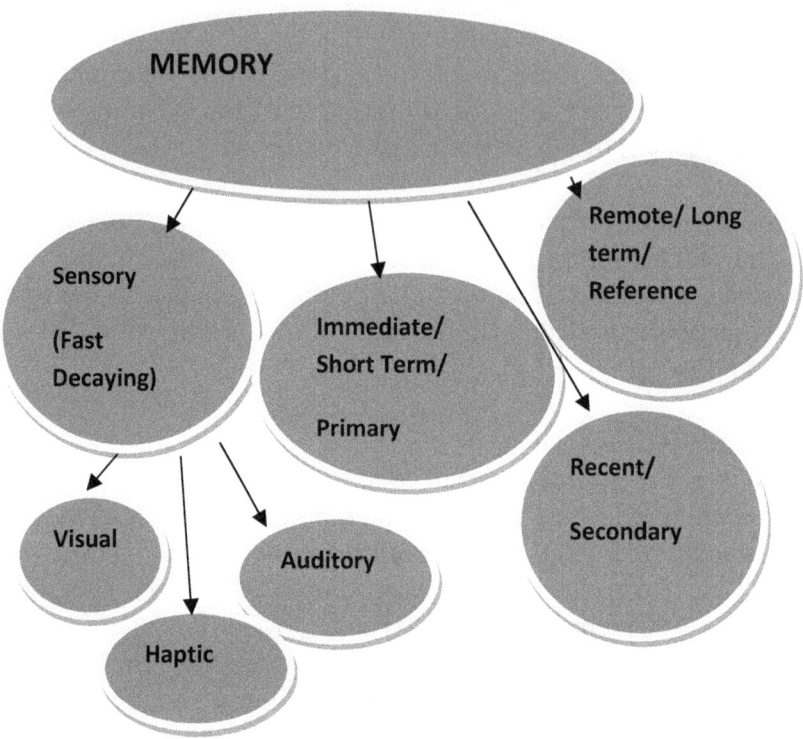

Fig 8: Classification of Memory Duration

Sensory Memory
This is fast decaying memory lasting in milliseconds to seconds. It could be visual (iconic mode) like after an image. It could be auditory (echoic); the bark of a dog or haptic (touch stimuli). The memory is uncertain because of the very fast duration.

Short term /Immediate Memory
Short term memory is the memory for events of few seconds or minutes. It has limited capacity of between five and nine numbers ($7_{\pm}2$) numbers. It is examined by asking the patient to repeat a sentence or a sequence of digits (Digit span). In examining for digit span, the examiner repeats numbers while the patient repeats after him. The examiner will increase the number of digits by one

sequentially e.g. say after me 342, he replies 342 then 2157 and he replies 2157 then continually increase the digits, 43528, 8563247. Most people should be able to repeat seven digits forward and five digits backwards. Chunking is the skill of splitting the number into smaller groups. It increases this limited capacity e.g. 0025-6742-9812-0534.This number which has a total of 16 digits has been split into chunks of 4 and memorized 4 at a time. In this manner, it is easy to commit 16 digits to memory.

Recent Memory/ Secondary memory
This is the memory of events that took place within weeks or months. It is tested with recent television events like a popular soap opera, the last meal or details of recent major events in the community, city or country. A person's accurate description of his illness during history taking is also a good test for recent memory.

Long term Memory/Remote/Reference
Long term memory is made up of past experiences. In assessing, asking about family accounts, personal issues and interests (marriages, births, deaths in the family, patient's education, jobs businesses) usually give better results and can be assessed while taking the history. The patient's accurate account of the history especially past medical history and coherence is a good assessment of his mental status. The long term memory is relatively resistant to the effects of neurological and psychiatric diseases hence patients with memory impairment may not remember very recent events but recall events that took places decades earlier with astounding clarity. The first name is everybody's earliest memory and is never lost. All neurological and psychiatric patients can speak still remember their first names. Long term memory can be reclassified according to the content. Other ways of classifying memory include

Memory According to Use
Working Memory
Episodic memory
Reference Memory

Memory According to Content

Memory according to content is actually a sub classification of long term memory.

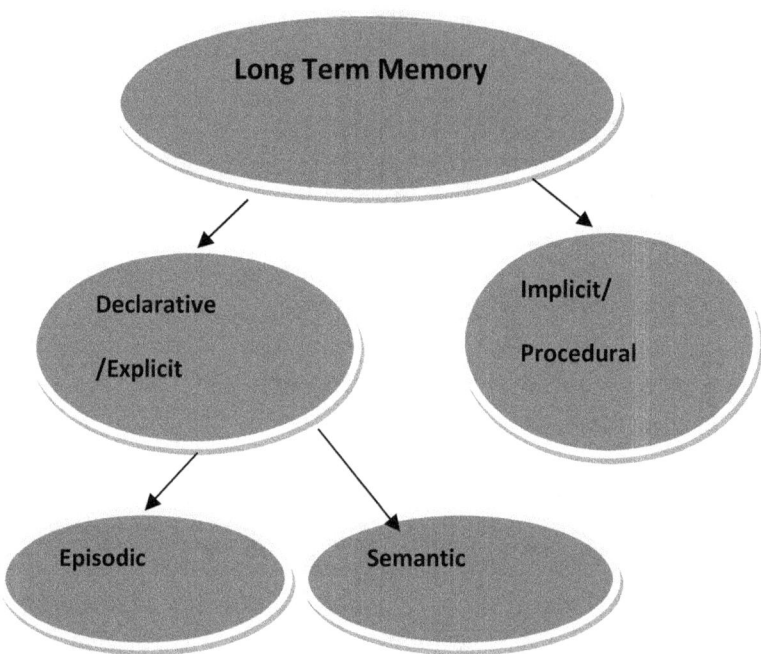

Fig 9: Classification of Memory according to content

Declarative memory (Knowing what)

This is the memory of facts and events that can be consciously retrieved. It is also called explicit memory. Declarative memory (limbic system) is further subdivided into two:

Episodic memory is the memory of autobiographical events (times, places, associated emotions, and other contextual who, what, when, where, why knowledge) that can be explicitly stated or conjured. It is therefore the collection of past personal experiences that occurred at a particular time and place. One characteristic of episodic memory is that it fades after a while in all normal persons. However, it can be reinforced by personal interest, novel, pleasant and traumatic experiences. Alzheimer's disease causes early loss of the episodic memory (early involvement of the limbic network).

Semantic
The second type is made up of all the unchanging facts, principles, associations and laws. These include unchanging facts like the days of the week, months of the years, countries and their capitals. It also includes unchanging principles, associations and laws like the physical attributes, colour of skin belong to a particular race, law of gravity, law of conception and others. In some cases, the semantic memory may also be episodic e.g. who was the President of Nigeria in the year 2017? It answers the question that starts with 'Who?' (Episodic) and it is also an unchanging fact (Semantic).

Non Declarative/ Procedural (knowing how)
Procedural (prefrontal cortex) memory is the unconscious memory of how to do things particularly the use of objects and how to do things. It is made up all acquired skills e.g. taking a bath, dressing, driving, sewing, cooking, surgical skills. They are performed with ease without conscious retrieval. Alzheimer's disease markedly affects the procedural memory such that the individual is unable to carry out procedures done with ease for many years; remember that it involves the prefrontal cortex later. One of the author's patients once came out of the bathroom without rinsing off the soap during a bath.

8.64 Loss of Executive function
Other cognitive operations impaired by prefrontal cortex lesions often are referred to as "executive functions." These are those cognitive and mental abilities that help people engage in goal-directed actions. They direct actions, control behaviour, and motivate individuals to achieve goals and prepare for future events. Components of the functions include the ability to manage time, pay attention and switch focus when there is need. It also includes the ability to plan, organize and remember details. Other components are the discretion to avoid saying or doing the wrong thing and the ability to do things based on past experience. Finally, executive function helps the individual to multitask. These functions are also badly impaired in Alzheimer's disease.

8.60 Emergence of primitive Reflexes

Primitive reflexes (frontal release signs, infantile or newborn reflexes) are seen at birth. They usually disappear in infancy as the brain develops. These reflexes however may reappear in adults due to certain neurological conditions. The re-emergence of these reflexes is commonly seen in persons with large structural lesions. This is especially in those that extend into the pre motor area of the frontal lobe. They are also seen in metabolic encephalopathies. However, the vast majority of patients with prefrontal lesions and frontal lobe behavioural syndromes do not display these reflexes. These reflexes are mediated by extrapyramidal functions, many of which are already present at birth.

They are however lost as the pyramidal tracts gain functionality with progressive myelination and development of the brain; usually disappearing at various times before the end of the first year of life. In fact most disappear within six months. *The absence of any of these reflexes in the newborn may indicate some neurological abnormality, local abnormality in the limb or neuromuscular disease.* Older children and adults with neurological disorders like cerebral palsy may retain these reflexes.. *Atypical primitive reflexes are also being researched as potential early warning signs of autistic spectrum disorders.*

8.70 Lesions of the hypothalamus and Pituitary

The diencephalon is the link between the nervous system and the endocrine system. The hypothalamus therefore controls the autonomic functions. A lot of autonomic disturbances arise from lesions of the hypothalamus. These include somnolence, problems with temperature regulation and obesity. Others are endocrine abnormalities like hypogonadism, hypothyroidism and Diabetes insipidus. Tumours of the pituitary (*the master gland*) have two special features; their numerous endocrine disturbances and their relationship to the optic chiasma. Compression of the optic chiasma produces the very rapid typical bitemporal hemianopia.

Disorders of the entorrhinal cortex may present with sleep disturbances. Circadian rhythm disorders are seen in lesions of the pineal gland.

8.80 Generalized Cortical lesions

These symptoms may arise from any aspect of the cerebral cortex. These are seizures, loss of consciousness, headaches, seizures and weakness. They may also be part of a more widespread systemic disease.

Seizures
Seizures are usually of cortical origin arising from any part of the cerebral cortex. A basic concept is that seizures may be either focal or generalized. Focal seizures originate from one cerebral hemisphere. They were once called partial seizures but the term *partial* is no longer used. Focal seizures are essential in localizing lesions because they are associated with structural abnormalities of the brain. Focal motor seizures with Jacksonian march, tonic eye and neck deviation indicate origin in the motor cortex. Haemorrhage and tumours may also cause focal seizures.

Generalized seizures however arise within and rapidly engage networks distributed across both cerebral hemispheres. They occur in diverse cellular, biochemical and structural abnormalities disorders especially infections and metabolic disturbances (hyperglycaemia, hypoglycaemia, renal and hepatic failure. Severe head trauma is one of the commonest causes of seizures in both adolescents and adults especially in cases of penetrating head wound, depressed skull fracture, intracranial haemorrhage, or subdural haematoma from an innocuous head trauma. Other causes of seizures include CVDs, CNS tumors, and degenerative diseases.

Loss of consciousness
A conscious state depends on intact cerebral hemispheres, the reticular activating system of the brain stem, hypothalamus and thalamus. Loss of consciousness is caused by damage to the RAS

or its projections, destruction of large portions of both cerebral hemispheres or suppression of reticulo-cerebral function by sepsis, drugs, toxins or metabolic derangements. Other common causes are intracerebral subarachnoid haemorrhage, trauma and brain stem strokes.

Headache
Headache is pain or discomfort between the orbits and occiput arising from pain sensitive structures. The intracranial pain sensitive structures are venous sinuses, cortical veins, basal arteries, dura of the anterior, middle and posterior fossae. The extracranial pain sensitive structures are scalp vessels and muscles, orbital contents, mucous membranes of the nasal and paranasal sinuses. Others are external and middle ear, teeth and gums. Pain can arise from the distortion, inflammation of these pain sensitive structures. Headache therefore can result from diverse aetiologies.

Weakness of the limbs

Movement is not a unique feature of the cortex. Brain stem, spinal cord, peripheral nerves and muscular lesions can cause weakness, so weakness of the limbs is not specific to the cerebral cortex. However, the weakness from hemispheric lesions classically involves one side of the body (face, upper and lower limbs) to varying degrees. When the brain stem is involved, there will be ipsilateral cranial nerve palsy and contralateral weakness (crossed paralysis). In general, if there is weakness, and the lesion is above the foramen magnum, then the site of the lesion causing the weakness is in the opposite brainstem or opposite hemisphere.

Weakness from a spinal lesion will not involve the face and it will be ipsilateral to the site of lesion. Weakness from the spinal cord and above (cortex, brain stem) will give the classical upper motor neurone features which include normal muscle bulk, hypertonia, hyperreflexia and extensor plantar response (spastic paralysis). Weakness from involving the anterior horn cell and below (peripheral nerves, neuromuscular junction and muscles) will give features of lower motor neurone lesions. These are wasting of muscles, fasciculations, hypotonia, hyporeflexia /areflexia and flexor plantar response (flaccid paralysis).

Cortical vs subcortical
Cortical lesions are lesions of the brain that affects the 4 lobes of the cerebral cortex (frontal, parietal, temporal and occipital lobes)
Sub cortical lesions are lesions that affect the structures in the subcortical area comprising mainly white matter (axons) like the internal capsule. The basal ganglia make up the grey matter (cell bodies or neurons) in the subcortical area.

Supratentorial vs Infratentorial
The tentorium cerebri is the part of the dura which separates the anterior and mid cranial fossae from the posterior fossa. Supratentorial structures are the structures above the tentorium cerebelli like the cortex, subcortical white matter and the basal ganglia. Infratentorial structures are the brainstem and cerebellum.

8.90 Common pathologies of the cerebral cortex

Cerebro Vascular Disorders
These are disorders that affect the vascular supply of the brain. Stroke, transient ischemic attack, aneurysms, and vascular malformations are all types of cerebrovascular disease. Other examples include a narrowing or blockage in the carotid, intracranial, or vertebral arteries, known as stenosis. Features of cerebrovascular diseases are diverse. Commonest is hemiparesis (weakness of one side face, upper and lower limbs). Other neurological features include hemi sensory loss, hemianopia, aphasia, apraxia and hemineglect.

Cerebral venous thrombosis
Cerebral venous sinus thrombosis (CVST) is the presence of acute thrombosis (a blood clot) in the dural venous sinuses. Symptoms may include headache, abnormal vision, any of the symptoms of stroke such as weakness of the face and limbs on one side of the body, and seizures.

Dementia
Dementia is actually not a specific disease. It's rather an overall term that describes a group of symptoms associated with a decline in memory and or other cognitive skills severe enough to impair a person's ability to perform everyday activities.

Infections
All the categories of infectious agents including bacteria, viruses, fungi, protozoa, and prion cause infections of the brain.

Metabolic
The *metabolic encephalopathies* are made up of a series of neurological disorders not caused by primary structural abnormalities; rather, they result from systemic illness, such as diabetes, liver disease, renal failure and heart failure

Toxins
Exposure to certain toxins causes toxic encephalopathies. Some of these include neurotoxic organic solvents such as toluene, heavy metals such as manganese or mercury. In some cases, there is an exposure to extreme concentrations of natural toxin such as cyanotoxins.

Neoplasia
Tumours of the brain may be primary or secondary. A primary *brain* tumor is a tumor which begins in the *brain* tissue while a secondary or metastatic lesion is a tumour that starts elsewhere in the body but spreads to the *brain*. Their features reflect the site of the tumour, the compression of adjacent structures and features of raised intracranial pressure.

References

1. Ekeh Bertha C; Clinical Neurology made Easy 1st Ed USA 2018
2. http://www.human-memory.net/types_declarative.html
3. Howlett Neurology in Africa Bergen, Norway 2012
4. Kasper DL, Fauci A S, Hauser S L, Longo D L, Jameson J L, Loscalzo J: Harrison's Principles of Internal Medicine; 19th Ed New York 2015
5. Lindsay K W. Bone I: Neurology and Neurosurgery Illustrated 4th Ed Edinburgh 2005
6. Ropper AH, Brown R H: Adams and Victor' Principles of Neurology 8th Ed New York 2005
7. Swash M, Glynn M: Hutchinson Clinical Methods 22nd Ed Edinburgh 2007
8. Zazulia A R. Neurological Diagnosis & Localization; https://neuro.wustl.edu/education/medical-student-education/neurology-clerkship/localization/

CHAPTER 9

LESIONS OF THE BASAL GANGLIA

8.0 Introduction

The basal ganglia (or basal nuclei) is made up of a group of subcortical nuclei. They are located at the base of the forebrain. They are well interconnected with the cerebral cortex, thalamus, and brainstem, as well as several other brain areas. Structures in the basal ganglia include the striatum, globus pallidus, substantia nigra, and the subthalamic nucleus. These structures are integral to voluntary motor function. Current research has shown that they are like a group of components of cortico-subcortical circuits, which originate in cortical areas, traverse the basal ganglia and terminate in specific areas in the frontal lobe. These areas are probably control not only motor function but also oculomotor, prefrontal, associative, and limbic functions. Diseases of the basal ganglia occur when these nuclei fail to properly suppress unwanted movements or to properly prime upper motor neuron circuits to initiate motor function. Understanding these circuits is very important in understanding the disorders of the basal ganglia.

9.10 Basal ganglia circuits

In order to excite the thalamus two distinct pathways are involved. These are the the direct and the indirect pathways. Most of the tracts as shown in Fig 10 are inhibitory; these have GABA as the neurotransmitter (red). The excitatory neurones are few: they are glutamatergic (purple). The dopaminergic neurones are modulatory (orange).

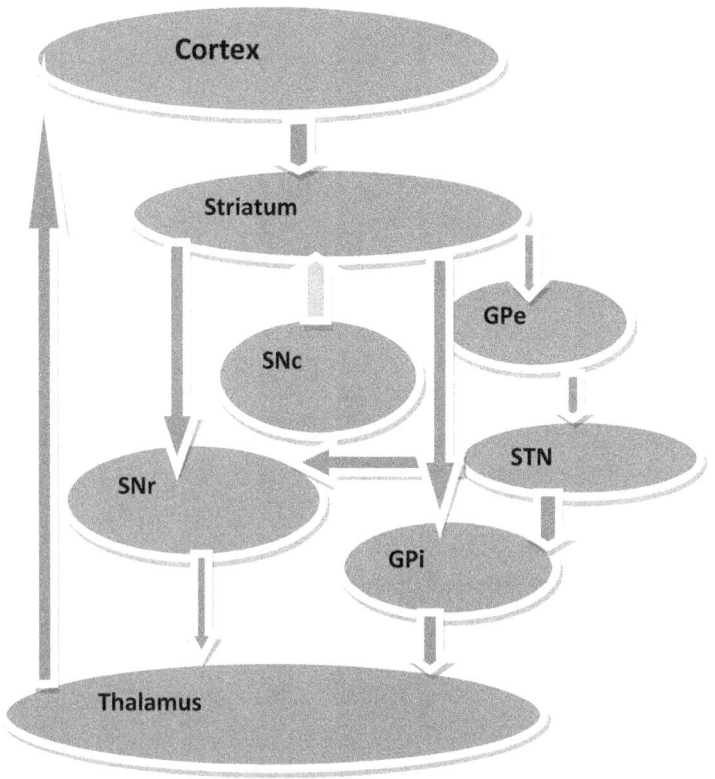

Fig 10 Connectivity diagram showing basal ganglia circuits

9.11 Direct pathway

9.11Direct pathway

The direct pathway of the motor circuit starts from the cortex. They move directly to the internal segment of the globus pallidus (GPi) or the substantia nigra pars reticulata (SNr) passing through the striatum. They eventually get to the thalamus and brainstem. This pathway initiates voluntary movements by exciting the thalamus which in turn excites the cortex. The excitation of the thalamus is achieved by disinhibiting the inhibitory neurones (double inhibition leads to excitation). This process is regulated by dopamine from the Substantia nigra pars compacta (SNc): the nigro- striatal pathway(orange) .

9.12 Indirect pathway

The indirect pathway of the motor circuit starts from the cerebral cortex to the thalamus and brainstem. It passes through the external segment of the globus pallidus (GPe) and the subthalamic nucleus (STN) indirectly. The STN is excited by the two-step inhibition (excitation) from the striatum. The STN then excites the internal segment of the globus pallidus (GPi) and the SNr which lead to the inhibition of the thalamus. There is therefore a termination of unwanted movements by this inhibition. *In essence, the excitation of the indirect pathway has the net effect of inhibiting thalamic neurons (rendering them unable to excite motor cortex neurons).* The indirect pathway is also regulated by dopamine released in the striatum; this is similar to the direct pathway. The inhibition at the striatum is through the D2 receptors. This is the inhibitory pathway. The red arrows are GABAergic neurones; they are inhibitory. All the purple arrows Glutamatergic neurones; they are excitatory. The modulatory nigro-striatal pathway on the other hand is dopaminergic (orange)

9.20 Extrapyramidal lesions

There is need for the balance of the two pathways to ensure the normal functioning of the basal ganglia. An upset of this balance results in the motor dysfunctions that characterize the **extrapyramidal disorders**. Excessive unmodulated basal ganglia output (reduction in Dopamine) causes inhibition of the thalamocortical projection neurons with subsequent difficulty in the initiation of voluntary movements. *These disorders are known as hypokinetic disorders.* When there is an interruption of the indirect pathway, there is reduction or absence of the inhibition of the thalamocortical projection neurons. This leads to an inability to suppress unwanted involuntary movements. *These disorders are known as hyperkinetic disorders.* The extrapyramidal tract's efferent fibers communicate via the cerebral cortex and thalamus and do not communicate directly with the spinal cord. *Hence in lesions to the Basal Ganglia, the patients have NO paresis or neuropsychological impairments.However, anthralgia and fatigue can mimic weakness.* Studies have shown that disorders of the basal ganglia can lead to other dysfunctions such as obsessive compulsive disorder (OCD) and Tourette syndrome.

9.30 Hypokinetic movement disorders

Excessive basal ganglia output as noted earlier is the cause of hypokinetic movement disorders. A common aetiology is the depletion of dopamine in the nigro striatal pathway. *These disorders are referred to as hypokinetic disorders.* The classical hypokinetic movement disorder is Parkinson disease.

Parkinson Disease

Classical features of Parkinson disease are varying degrees of: (1) rigidity, (2) bradykinesia, (3) tremor, and (4) postural abnormalities. Rigidity is present in all ranges of passive manipulation and active movement. This is due to an over activity in descending motor pathways from the brain stem. Rigidity is elicited on the hinge joints where both flexion and extension movements are rigid; lead pipe rigidity (like attempting to bend or straighten a lead pipe). The rigidity also accounts to some extent the flexed posture seen in Parkinson disease. In association with tremors, the rigidity takes on cogwheel character (like a chain moving on the cogs or teeth of a wheel).

Bradykinesia

In bradykinesia (reduced movements), there is an inability to initiate or carry out voluntary movements despite the presence of adequate strength. Observable features include an absence or reduction of facial expressions, fidgeting, gesticulations or arm swinging while walking. The absence of facial expressions causes a masked face. The patient sits like a statue and does not fidget in any way like adjusting the tie, the hair or cross the legs. The patient however retains the ability to carry out motivated, well learned and automatic behaviours. *Bradykinesia is considered the most disabling feature of Parkinson disease.*

Bradykinesia usually co-exists with rigidity and the additive effect is immobilizing. Such persons appear frozen. Rarely, there may be a small number of patients that have only bradykinesia without the rigidity or tremors. This is noted to be a pure "ignition" syndrome.

Tremors

Tremors are rhythmic oscillations of opposing muscle groups. The movements are two-way movements (flexion –extension, pronation-supination, left–right, up-down, open-close). The tremors involve the extremities but may also involve the neck, head, lips and tongue. The frequency of the tremor in Parkinson disease is 4-8/sec, affects the upper extremities earlier than the lower extremities and does not involve the head. Typically the Parkinson tremor starts from one side of the body before involving the other side of the body. It is also worse at rest and characteristically seen with the hands folded in the lap. It is however suppressed by the initiation of voluntary movement. The tremors like other involuntary movements disappear at rest. Postural deficits albeit not well studied and understood are also seen in Parkinson disease. The combination of rigidity and bradykinesia leaves the patient frozen. The flexed stooped posture (Simian posture) is considered a compensation for the postural imbalance. There is great difficulty in adjusting to postural changes like catching their balance. A simple shove or even looking up will make the person fall like a tree instead of catching his balance.

9.40 Hyperkinetic movement Disorders

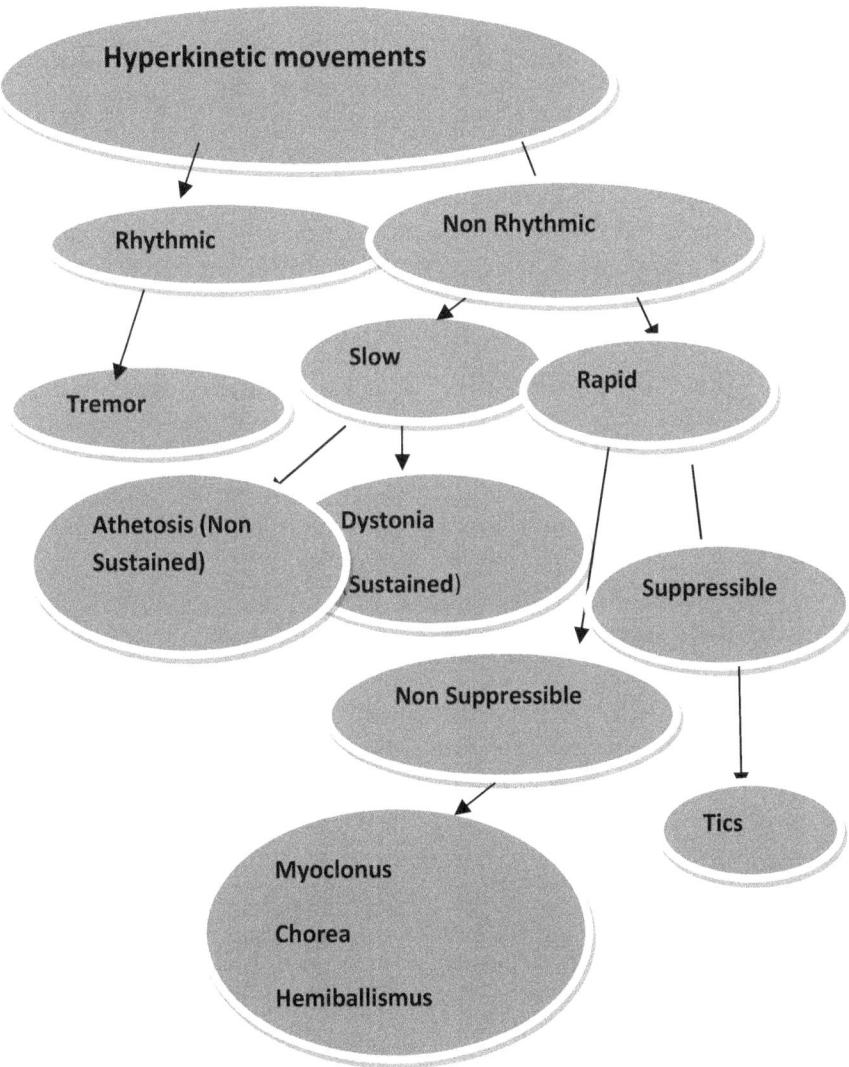

Fig 11: Classification of hyperkinetic movements

9.41 Rhythmic hyperkinetic movements

Tremors are the only rhythmic of the all the movements.

9.42 Tremors

Tremors as described above are the most common of the involuntary movements and are seen in hyperkinetic movement disorders. They are oscillations of one or more body parts like the hands, arms, eyes, head, vocal folds, trunk, and legs. Most tremors however occur in the hands.

Physiological tremors

Tremors are not always symptoms of a neurological disorder. Physiological tremor occurs in every normal individual and has no clinical significance. It is rarely visible and may be heightened by strong emotion (such as anxiety or fear), physical exhaustion, hypoglycaemia, hyperthyroidism, stimulants, alcohol withdrawal or fever. Physiological tremors may be observed in all voluntary muscle groups. Clinically, this is detected by tremors the shaking of the a piece of paper placed on top of an extended hand. Commonly seen physiological tremor is the chattering of the teeth. This may be caused by cold temperatures or by fear. Rigors from malarial fever also cause tremulousness.Occasionally the physiological tremor is enhanced to more visible levels with a frequency of 10Hz which is caused by a reaction to certain drugs, alcohol withdrawal, or medical conditions including an overactive thyroid and hypoglycaemia. Heightened emotion, stress, fever, physical exhaustion, or low sugar may trigger tremors or increase their severity These are reversible once the cause is corrected.

Psychogenic tremor (also called hysterical tremor)

This type of tremor can occur at rest, postural or when in motion. Characteristics vary but commonly include sudden onset and remission, increased incidence with stress. There is an unusual occurrence of the tremors to change in direction or a change in the part of the body affected. Typically, the tremor is greatly decreased or may totally disappear when the patient is distracted. Persons with psychogenic tremor have a conversion disorder or another psychiatric disease

9.43 Types of Pathologic Tremors

Traditionally tremors are classified into three types. These are

Intention tremor

Intention tremors are slow, broad and affect the extremities. They usually occur at the end of a purposeful movement. This includes trying to button a shirt or touching a finger to the tip of one's nose. Such a person will notice that his glass of water or spoon of food spills with a change in the person's writing. Intention tremor is classically seen in cerebellar disorders and at such it is also called cerebellar tremor.

Rest Tremors

Rest tremors are maximal at rest and become less prominent with activity. They are best seen when the patient is seated with the hands folded. The tremor is usually coarse and affects distal limbs usually the hands with a rate of 3-8 Hertz (cycles/second). They usually occur as an isolated symptom or often a precursor to Parkinson's disease. The tremor, which is classically seen as a "pill-rolling" action (It looks like the person is rolling a pill in between the fingers) of the hands. There may also be affectation of the chin, lips, legs, and trunk.

Postural Tremors/Orthostatic tremor

Postural tremors are maximal when the limb is actively maintained against gravity. In essence, they occur immediately after standing. They are less when the person is at rest. In addition voluntary movement towards a target does not enhance the tremors. The frequency of the tremors is > 12/Hz; hence they are fast as well as fine. Such a person will shake uncontrollably on standing one a spot. There are associated cramps in the thighs and legs. The shaking and cramp cease once the person sits. The patient will not have any other clinical symptoms or signs. The high frequency of the tremor often makes it look like rippling of leg muscles while standing. These tremors may co exist in persons with essential tremor. In some cases, the hands are most often affected but the head, voice, tongue, legs, and trunk may also be involved. Head tremor occasionally present in a vertical (repeated nodding) way called titubation, or horizontal motion (No-No tremors).

9.44 Other types of Tremors

Rubral tremor is associated with conditions which affect the red nucleus in the midbrain, classically unusual strokes. It is characterized by coarse slow tremor which is present at rest, at posture and with intention.

Peripheral Neuropathy Tremors

Tremors also occur in cases of peripheral neuropathy. This may manifest as a tremor or ataxia of the affected limbs and problems with gait and balance. Clinical characteristics may be similar to features of essential tremor which are postural.

Dystonic tremors

Dystonic tremor occurs in individuals who have dystonia. Dystonic tremors occur in all muscles of the body and generally affect muscles in certain positions. The pattern of dystonic tremor may differ from essential tremor. They occur irregularly and can be relieved by complete rest in most cases. Typically, touching the affected body part or muscle may reduce tremor severity (a geste antagoniste). The tremor may be the initial sign of dystonia localized to a particular part of the body.

9.50 Non Rhythmical involuntary movements

All other involuntary movements are non-rhythmical and are classified according to their speed, part of the body involved and ability to be suppressed voluntary control.

9.51 Slow movements

Athetosis

Athetosis is a rare slow movement disorder. It is characterized by involuntary, slow, twisting, writhing (moves like an earthworm) movements. The movements occur nearly continuously in distal muscles being most pronounced in the digits, hands, face and tongue. There is an inability to sustain the fingers, toes, or tongue in one position. Striatal injury, particularly prominent in the putamen, has been considered the site of injury. The most common cause is perinatal hyperbilirubinemia to developing forebrain with cortical and prominent basal ganglia damage. Athetosis in these cases is often associated erratic choreiform components; choreo-athetoid movements.

Dystonia/Torsion Spasm

Dystonia is a movement disorder in which sustained involuntary muscle contractions cause twisting and repetitive motions and or painful with abnormal postures or positions. Dystonia overlaps with athetosis. It is produced by co contraction of agonists and antagonist muscles that place the limb in an unnatural position. It may take the form of overextension/overflexion, as well as inversion/eversion of the foot. There may also be torsion of the spine, forced eye closure (blepharospasm) or a fixed grimace. Dystonias may be progressive or static and are related to past encephalitis in a few cases but are usually idiopathic. Dystonia is caused by various combinations of basal ganglia lesions. The commonest form is spasmodic torticollis which is characterized by intermittent excessive and involuntary contractions of the sternocleidomastoid muscle on one side. On rare occasions, the contraction of the sternocleidomastoid may be bilateral. This is called retrocollis. Antecollis also occurs when there is excessive involuntary leading to a forward bending of the neck. Commonly, dystonias result from overdose of Neuroleptic drugs. This is always reversible when the drug is withdrawn or counteracted by Anticholinergic drugs. Involuntary and occasionally severe tonic contraction of axial muscles is most common, ranging from jaw clenching similar to the trismus (lockjaw) of tetanus to severe opisthotonic posturing (back and neck in sustained extension) similar to that seen in decerebration.

9.52 Rapid movements

Tics

Tics are certain movements which are of no purpose. They may be complex or simple and are usually momentary. They often occur repetitively in a single location and sometimes multifocal. They are the only involuntary movements that can be suppressed for sometime by voluntary control. Tics may be confused with fasciculations and myokymia. Fasciculations are usually elicited mechanically and occur in lower motor neurone lesion hence there is associated weakness and wasting of muscles. Myokymia often occurs after fatigue e.g. the eye muscles after sleepless nights. Tics are common and usually transient in children (often brought on by stress, which worsens all tic disorders). However, some children have multiple motor tics and repetitive vocal tics (throat clearing, snorting, sniffing, etc) which are features of Tourette syndrome. Vocal tics may become so severe that the words may include expletives (coprolalia). These symptoms may resolve or persist into adulthood. Tics in children may be accompanied by symptoms of obsessive-compulsive disorder and Attention deficit/Hyperactive Disorder (ADHD) (psycho stimulants used to treat ADHD usually worsen tics).

Myoclonus

Myoclonus is a brief, involuntary twitching or jerking of a muscle or a group of muscles. They are caused by sudden muscle contractions (*positive myoclonus*) or brief lapses of contraction (*negative myoclonus*). Myoclonic jerks can be physiological or pathological. Physiological myoclonic jerks is the sudden drop of the head in a person who is feeling sleepy. They are also called hypnic jerks and occur in all human beings. Myoclonic jerks therefore occur in healthy persons but are pathological when they become persistent and widespread. The myoclonic jerk of the diaphragm is also called hiccups. Asterixis which have been erroneously termed flappy tremors are actually myoclonic jerks. Myoclonic jerks may occur singularly or as part of a sequence. They may also occur in a pattern or without pattern. Commonest cause of myoclonic jerks are metabolic disorders like hyperglycaemic hyperosmolar state (HHS), uraemic encephalopathy, electrolyte imbalances and infections. ***In fact just like physiological myoclonus is seen in persons about to fall into a physiologic sleep, pathological myoclonus is usually seen in persons about to fall into a pathologic sleep (coma).*** Neurological causes of myoclonus include multiple sclerosis, Parkinson's disease, Dystonia, Alzheimer's disease, Gaucher's disease, subacute sclerosing panencephalitis, Creutzfeldt–Jakob disease (CJD), serotonin toxicity, some cases of Huntington's disease, some forms of epilepsy, and occasionally in intracranial hypotension. It is therefore important to differentiate between myoclonic jerks and myoclonic seizures. *The most important difference is the level of consciousness.* In persons with myoclonic seizures, consciousness is impaired. On the other hand, consciousness is usually preserved in myoclonic jerks. However, the person with myoclonic jerks may eventually lapse into unconsciousness if the cause is not treated.

Chorea

Chorea is derived from the same word as choreography; it means "dance". It is a type of involuntary movement disorder characterized by irregular and fleeting movements of the limbs and/or axial musculature also including the muscles of the face, jaw and tongue. The intensity of movement has a very wide range of variation (from mild buccal movements t o exhaustive flailing). In fact, chorea is considered a milder form of hemiballismus. In chorea, the abnormal movements affect more of the lower limbs; this makes it look like a dance. Hemiballismus on the other hand affects more of the upper limbs. Degenerative and destructive processes in the striatum or striatal inhibition by drugs are the commonest causes of chorea. The prototype choreiform disorder is Huntington's chorea. This is a rare, inherited (autosomal dominant), degenerative disorder. The pathological process involves the striatum, as well as the cerebral cortex. The clinical presentation is a triad of involuntary movements (chorea), dementia and psychiatric disturbances. Huntington's chorea is an incurable disease. Sydenham's or rheumatic chorea is a mild, self-limited limb and axial disorder associated with rheumatic fever in children. Other causes are pregnancy (chorea gravidarum), oral contraceptive pills, hyperthyroidism and rarely SLE. Medications that may cause chorea include atropine poisoning, anticonvulsant toxicity (e.g., Phenytoin, Carbamazepine, and Phenobarbital), and L-dopa.

Hemiballismus

Hemiballismus is the most rapid of all the abnormal involuntary movements. It is a violent flinging movement of the limb usually the arm. It is classically a unilateral lesion hence the "hemi". Rarely these abnormal movements may be bilateral (bilateral ballismus). It is caused by a lesion in the contralateral subthalamic nucleus or, rarely, the striatum. An infarct is the commonest aetiology and less often haemorrhage, and rarely tumour.

9.60 Tardive dyskinesia

Tardive dyskinesia(i.e.dyskinesias appearing late) is characterized by repetitive, involuntary movements that appear after long term neuroleptic use : *tardive dyskinesia is medication induced.* It is made up of rapid involuntary movements usually involving the lips and face. Some of these include grimacing, tongue movements, lip smacking, puckering and pursing. There may be excessive blinking. Occasionally, there may be affectation of the limbs, torso, and fingers. *Unlike Parkinson disease in which patients have difficulty moving, persons with tardive dyskinesia patients have difficulty not moving.* Affectation of the trunk muscles causes a characteristic irregular pelvic thrusting movement. In severe cases, there is a feeling of inner restlessness and a compelling need to be in constant motion. The range of movement includes the following: rocking while standing or sitting, lifting the feet repeatedly as though he is marching on the spot as well as crossing and uncrossing the legs while sitting. This is referred to as akathisia. Tardive dyskinesia occurs as a result compensatory increase in the number of dopamine receptor sites following long-term administration of neuroleptic drugs, producing hypersensitivity.

References

1. Baliga R R: 250 short cases in clinical Medicine 3rd Ed Saunders 2001.
2. Ekeh Bertha C; Clinical Neurology made Easy 1st Ed USA 2018
3. https://en.wikipedia.org/wiki/Basal_ganglia_disease
4. Howlett. Neurology in Africa Bergen, Norway 2012
6. Kasper DL, Fauci A S, Hauser S L, Longo D L, Jameson J L, Loscalzo J: Harrison's Principles of Internal Medicine; 19th Ed New York 2015
7. Lindsay K W. Bone I: Neurology and Neurosurgery Illustrated 4th Ed Edinburgh 2005
9. Ropper AH, Brown R H: Adams and Victor' Principles of Neurology 8th Ed New York 2005
10. Swash M, Glynn M: Hutchinson Clinical Methods 22nd Ed Edinburgh 2007
11. Walker HK, Hall WD, Hurst JW; Clinical Methods, The History, Physical, and Laboratory Examinations 3rd Ed Boston 1990
12. University of Texas: Neuroscience online, an electronic textbook for NeuroSciences

CHAPTER 10

LESIONS OF THE POSTERIOR FOSSA

10.10 Lesions of The of Brainstem

The brainstem is a crowded location where most motor and sensory pathways travel on their way to other locations since the brain stem plays a major role in conduction. All the pathways both ascending and descending traverse through the brain stem to and fro the cerebral cortex, spinal cord and cerebellum. In addition, there are upper motor neurons that originate in the brainstem's vestibular, red, tectal, and reticular nuclei, which also descend and synapse in the spinal cord. Lesions of the brainstem often involve loss of blood supply or tumors, which typically occur in restricted areas or quadrants and involve adjacent structures (neighbors!) of multiple systems.

The second important function of the brainstem is the emergence of cranial nerves three to twelve from the brainstem. These cranial nerves supply the face, head, and viscera. The brainstem also has integrative functions being involved in cardiovascular system control and respiratory control.

Finally, the brain stem through the reticular activating formation plays a major role pain sensitivity control, alertness, awareness, and consciousness.

Lesions of the brain stem therefore will present with features of the affected tract which ranges from changes in sensory deficits, muscle weakness, involuntary movements to difficulty in co-ordination. Others are cranial nerve abnormalities, the dreaded cardio-respiratory collapse and loss of consciousness. Localizing the brain stem lesion is considered one of the most challenging aspects. A useful guide is the "Rules of 4" which simplifies the site of the tracts and the structures.

10.11 Rules of 4

The rules are summarized as follows:
1. **4 Structures in the midline: they all begin with "M"**
2. **4 Structures at the side: they all begin with "S"**

3. 4 Motor Nuclei in the midline: they are all divisors of 12(3rd, 4th, 6th and 12th)
4. 4 Cranial nerves in the medulla, 4 in the pons and 4 above the pons

10.12 The four midline structures
Motor pathway (corticospinal/pyramidal tract)
The corticospinal tract generally controls voluntary movement of the opposite side. This is due to the decussation in the medulla as it descends. Lesions of the corticospinal tract in the brainstem will lead to weakness of the opposite side of the body (*contralateral* hemiparesis) as seen in cortical lesions.

Medial lemniscus
This is part of the posterior column-medial lemniscus pathway. The posterior columns ascend in the posterior part of the spine to the brainstem. At the medulla, they *decussate* and synapse. The fibres pass to the thalamus and finally relay in the sensory cortex. The posterior columns convey sensory fibres which subserve fine touch and proprioception (joint position sense) and vibration. Damage will lead to *contralateral loss* of joint position sense and vibration.

Medial longitudinal fasciculus (MLF)
MLF is the main central connection for the occulomotor nerve, trochlear nerve, and abducens nerve. It is a myelinated tract that allows conjugate eye movement by connecting the paramedian pontine reticular formation (PPRF)-abducens nucleus complex of the contralateral side in the pons to the occulomotor nucleus of the ipsilateral side in the midbrain. Thus, the abducens nucleus contains interneurons that project via the medial longitudinal fasciculus to the medial rectus subnucleus of the contralateral occulomotor complex.This connection leads to lateral conjugate gaze (movement of the ipsilateral lateral rectus and the contralateral medial rectus).

Internuclei Ophthalmoplegia (INO)
Damage to the MLF cuts off the inter neurone to the 3rd nerve. This leads to lateral conjugate gaze disorder where there is diplopia as well as difficulty in adduction (medial rectus function) of the

affected eye. This referred to as inter nuclear ophthalmoplegia (INO); also called ataxic nystagmus. It is common in multiple sclerosis.

Other associated recognized MLF lesions are:
Webino syndrome (Wall eyes)
This is caused by bilateral damage to the MLF thereby causing bilateral internuclei ophthalmoplegia. This results in extropia and loss of convergence (bilateral medial nerve dysfunction).

One and a half syndrome
In this unusual syndrome, one eye cannot move laterally at all, while the other can only move in one lateral direction (outward). This is because there is conjugate horizontal gaze palsy (lesion of ipsilateral PPRF or 6th nerve nucleus) in one direction and an internuclear ophthalmoplegia (ipsilateral lesion of the MLF) in the other. The only remaining horizontal movement is contralateral abduction. Nystagmus is also present. When there is an association of the 7th nerve palsy, it is called eight and half syndrome.

Motor nuclei and nerves
The cranial nerve nuclei that are in the midline are those that are divisors of number 12. These are cranial nerves 3rd (occulomotor nerve nucleus), 4th (trochlear nerve nucleus), 6th (abducens nerve nucleus) and 12th (hypoglossal nerve nucleus). Damage to any of these cranial nerves will lead to *ipsilateral* since only the lower part of the face(7th and 12th) have inputs from the contralateral cortex) weakness of the muscles supplied by the cranial nerve. The nuclei of the other cranial nerves are *laterally* located in the brainstem.

10.13 The four structures to the side

Spinocerebellar tract
Both the anterior and posterior spinocerebellar tracts ascend on the same side of the cord and enter the cerebellum through the inferior and superior cerebellar peduncles respectively: they are *uncrossed* tracts. Damage to this tract causes *ipsilateral* ataxia.

Spinothalamic tracts

The lateral and anterior spinothalamic tracts bearing pain and temperature fibres enter the posterior roots, ascend a few segments and then *cross* to the opposite side (in the spine). In the spine, they ascend in these tracts to the thalamus, where they are relayed to the sensory cortex. Damage to the spinothalamic tracts causes *contralateral* pain and temperature loss.

Sensory nucleus of Trigeminal nerve

The processes arising from the trigeminal ganglion cells enter the lateral aspect of the pons. Here, they divide into ascending and descending branches. These branches terminate in one or other component of the sensory nucleus of V. The different parts of the nucleus subserves different sensory modalities viz touch, pain, temperature and proprioception. Damage to this nucleus causes *ipsilateral* loss of pain and temperature on the face.

Sympathetic chain

The sympathetic chain ascends deep inside the posterior wall of the carotid sheath. It follows this part till it reaches the base of the skull. The fibres which cause the dilatation of the pupillary muscle travel in this plexus beside the internal carotid artery. Grey rami pass from the superior ganglion to cranial nerves 7th, 9th, 10th and 12th. Damage of the sympathetic chain will cause to *ipsilateral* Horner's syndrome also called occulo sympathetic paresis. The features of Horner's syndrome are a classic triad of meiosis (constricted pupil), partial ptosis, and loss of hemi facial sweating (anhidrosis).

10.14 Nuclei of the cranial nerves in the brain stem

Four of cranial nuclei are located above the pons. These are the Olfactory (1st), Optic(2nd), Occulomotor (3rd) and trochlear (4th) nerves. The nuclei of the olfactory (1st) and optic (2nd) nerves are located in the cerebral cortex. The nuclei of the occulomotor and trochlear nerves lie in the midbrain.

Four other cranial nerve nuclei are located in the pons. These are trigeminal, abducens, facial and Vestibulocochlear (cranial nerves 5th -8th).

The last **four cranial nerve nuclei are located in the medulla**. These are glossopharyngeal, vagus, accessory and hypoglossal (cranial nerves 9th -12th). Damage to the cranial nerves will present with cranial nerve palsies depending of which cranial nerve is affected. These could be visual disturbances and double vision (Diplopia), difficulty in swallowing (Dysphagia), difficulty in phonation and voice change (Dysphonia). Others are difficulty in articulation of speech (Dysarthria) and hearing difficulty (Dysacusis): '**All the Ds**'.

Cranial nerve lesions have given rise to many syndromes that are crammed over the years by medical students and medical doctors. A simple method to localize these disorders is to note the following;

1. The cranial nerve involvement indicates the *horizontal level* of the lesion: midbrain, pons or medulla. Note the site of the nuclei of the nerves as described above. In essence, involvement of the 9th-12th nerve localizes the lesion to the medulla. Involvement of 5th -8th localizes it to the pons while involvement of 3rd or 4th indicates the midbrain. The involvement of the 1st or 2nd will localize the lesion to the cerebral cortex.
2. The involvement of the tract indicates the *vertical axis* of the lesion whether it is in the midline or in the lateral aspect of the spine.

There are structures in the midline and on the side as noted above. Hence hemiparesis, loss of vibration and joint position sense, internuclei ophthalmoplegia and palsy of the midline cranial nerves indicate that the lesion is in the midline. In the same vein, ataxia, loss of pain and temperature, loss of sensation over the face and Horner's syndrome will indicate a lesion on the side.

Some authors have described it as *latitudes* (nerves) and *longitudes* (tracts).

10.15 Brain Stem syndromes (eponymic syndromes)
The following are midbrain lesions.

Lesions of the midbrain
The involvement of the occulomotor nerve indicates that the horizontal level is at the *midbrain*. These lesions result in some classic syndromes as follows;

Nothnagel's syndrome
There is ipsilateral occulomotor palsy and contralateral cerebellar ataxia. It is caused by damage to the superior cerebellar peduncle; a structure in the midbrain that is near the third nerve. The superior cerebellar peduncle has *crossed* fibres hence the deficit is contralateral.

Benedikt's syndrome
There is ipsilateral occulomotor palsy and contralateral tremor, chorea, and athetosis. This is caused by injury to the red nucleus. Fibres from the red nucleus *cross* at the medulla.

Claude's syndrome
There are features of both Nothnagel's and Benedikt's syndromes. This is caused by injuries to both the red nucleus and the superior cerebellar peduncle.

Weber's syndrome
There is ipsilateral occulomotor palsy with contralateral hemiparesis. This is caused by an injury to the cerebral peduncle.

Parinaud's syndrome
Parinaud's syndrome is also known as dorsal midbrain syndrome, vertical gaze palsy, or Sunset Sign. In this syndrome, there is an inability to move the eyes up and down. It is caused by compression of the vertical gaze center at the rostral interstitial nucleus of medial longitudinal fasciculus (riMLF). The slightly dilated pupils react on accommodation but not to light (light-near dissociation).

Lesions of the Pons
The occurrence of ipsilateral 6th nerve palsy localizes the horizontal level of the lesions to the pons.

Foville's syndrome
There is ipsilateral gaze palsy, ipsilateral facial palsy, and contralateral hemiparesis. This is caused dorsal pontine injury in the midline (the corticospinal tract and 6th nerve nucleus are mid line structures).

Millard-Gubler syndrome
Millard-Gubler syndrome is similar to Foville's however there is only lateral rectus weakness, instead of the complete lateral gaze palsy. It occurs from injury to the ventral pons which involves only the abducens fascicle rather than the nucleus. Infarct, tumour, haemorrhage, vascular malformation, and multiple sclerosis are the most common aetiologies of brainstem abducens palsy.

Locked in State
The locked in state is most often due to a lesion in the ventral pons (basis pontis). Commonest aetiology is the occlusion of the basilar artery or haemorrhage into the ventral pons which transects all the descending corticospinal and corticobulbar pathways. It is characterized by inability to produce speech or volitional movements despite being awake. The person is unable to indicate that he is awake but vertical eye movements and the elevation of the lids remains intact. This is because the midbrain elements that allow the eyelids to be raised are also spared. Hence such a person is able to communicate with vertical gaze and blinking. There is also sparing of both the somatosensory pathways and the ascending neuronal systems responsible for arousal and wakefulness. Severe motor neuropathy like in Guillian Barre syndrome, pontine myelinosis or periodic paralysis may give a similar picture. Other causes are critical illness neuropathy and pharmacologic neuromuscular blockade.

Lesions of the Medulla

Medullary Syndromes are characteristic because of the decussation of different tracts and the nerves that run through them. Two recognized syndromes will be discussed here.
They are Lateral Medullary Syndrome (Wallenberg's syndrome) and the medial medullary syndrome.

Wallenberg Syndrome/Lateral medullary syndrome
This syndrome is caused by infarct of the lateral medulla supplied by the posterior inferior cerebellar arteries. The features reflect the damage to the tracts or structures involved as follows: ipsilateral loss of pain and temperature sensation over one-half of the face (sensory nucleus of the trigeminal tract). There is ipsilateral ataxia (spinocerebellar tract), nystagmus diplopia, vertigo, nausea and vomiting (vestibular nucleus). Others are Horner's syndrome (descending sympathetic tract) and dysphagia, hoarseness, paralysis of the palate and vocal cord, diminished gag reflex (9th, 10th) nerves and loss of taste (Nucleus of the tractus solitarius). Finally there is contralateral loss of pain and temperature sense over half the body (Spinothalamic tract).

Medial medullary syndrome
This arises from occlusion of vertebral artery supplying the medial medulla. Features are ipsilateral paralysis with atrophy of one-half half the tongue (12th nerve) and contralateral paralysis of arm and leg, sparing face; impaired tactile and proprioceptive sense over one-half the body (pyramidal tract and medial lemniscus).

10.16 Lesions of the Reticular Formation

Sleep and consciousness
The reticular formation is very important in establishing states of consciousness like alertness and sleep. Injury to the reticular formation can result in irreversible coma. In fact the state of irreversible brain damage where all the brain stem reflexes are absent is considered death.

Cardiovascular control
Affectation of the vital centers and reticular activating system will lead to loss of consciousness, cardiovascular and respiratory collapse.

Loss of somatic motor control
There will be difficulty in maintenance of balance and posture during body movements.

10.17 Other lesions of the brain stem are;
Brainstem herniation
The cranium is a closed cavity. In cases of raised intracranial pressure the brainstem can herniated through the foramen magnum (coning) thereby compressing the vital respiratory and circulatory centres. This is a fatal complication which necessitates urgent surgical decompression (either with Burr hole or trepanning). In trepanning; segments of the skull are removed to relieve pressure.

10.20 Lesions of the Cerebellum

Parts of the cerebellum

Archicerebellum (vestibulocerebellum): It includes the flocculonodular lobe, which is located in the medial zone. The archicerebellum helps maintain equilibrium and coordinate eye, head, and neck movements; it is closely interconnected with the vestibular nuclei.

Midline vermis (paleocerebellum): It helps coordinate trunk and leg movements. Vermis lesions result in abnormalities of stance and gait.

Lateral hemispheres (neocerebellum): They control quick and finely coordinated limb movements, predominantly of the arms.

10.21 Ataxia

Ataxia is made up of the lack of voluntary control of movements leading to the disorderliness of the movements and gait. Cerebellar tremor arises from impairment of the smooth coordination of ongoing movements and motor planning. It is a core feature of lesions of the cerebellum though absent in some cerebellar lesions. There is difficulty in regulating the force, range, direction, velocity and rhythm of muscle contractions. The result is a characteristic type of irregular, uncoordinated movement. Manifestations include abnormal physical weakness or lack of energy (*asthenia*) and difficulty in coordination between muscles or limbs that usually act in unison (*asynergy*). Other features are delayed reaction time, and a distorted perception in time (*dyschronometria*). People with cerebellar ataxia may initially present with poor balance. This is seen as an inability to stand on one leg or perform the tandem walk. Tandem walk is the ability to walk on a straight line placing one foot before the other. As the condition progresses, there is the characteristic *cerebellar ataxic gait* which is also called the drunken sailor gait. It is a broad based gait. Typically, the patient's feet are wide apart. The patient is unable to put his feet together and is unsteady.There is also an erratic shifting of weight from one side to the other. The person also finds it difficult to turn and attempts to turn results in falls.

10.22 Holmes Rebound phenomenon

The rebound phenomenon is also known as the *loss of the check reflex*. It is a reflex that occurs on attempting to move a limb against resistance. On sudden removal of the resistance, the limb should move a short distance in the original direction at first. Thereafter, the antagonist muscles will contract, causing the muscle to yank back in the opposite direction. In essence the antagonistic muscles place a *check* on the movement. This check is strongly exaggerated in upper motor neurone lesions where there is spasticity. In cerebellar dysfunction however the limb continues moving in the same direction; the check by the antagonist muscles is absent.

10.23 Dysarthria

Another feature of cerebellar dysfunction is dysarthria (impairment in articulation). The speech is made up of a slower irregular rhythm with variable volume. The patient seems to place equal and excessive stress on all syllabi spoken (*scanning or staccato speech*). There may also be slurring of speech with associated tremors of the voice. The voice quality may be harsh and the loudness varies excessively to a degree that it may become *explosive* because of the increased effort. Hyper nasality is not common but may occur.

10.24 Dysdiadokinesia

Dysdiadochokinesia is taken from three words: *dys* (bad), *diadocho* (succeeding) *kinesia* (movement). There is difficulty in rapidly alternating movements. This is usually examined by the rapid alternation of pronation and supination of the forearm which should be rhythmic (two-way). These movements will be disorderly and lack the usual rhythm.

10.25 Dysmetria
Dysmetria (optic ataxia) refers to difficulty with distances and lengths. The patient has an inability to judge distances or ranges of movement. This may be seen as undershooting, (*hypometria),* or overshooting, (*hypermetria). In hypometria, the patient is unable to reach the required target while he overshoots the target in hypermetria.* The person therefore will be noted to bang objects on the table or hit walls on parking his car because he had misjudged the distance. Dysmetria is elicited with the finger –nose test or heel –shin test. The patient will either overshoot (past pointing/hypermetria) or undershoot (hypometria). Dysmetria worsens with increasing speed.

Hypotonia
Mild decrease in the tone of muscles is a feature of cerebellar disease.

10.26 Intention Tremor

There is a rhythmic oscillatory movement of the limb as it reaches towards a target. It is coarse and broad. Intention tremor may also involve the head and eyes as well as the limbs and torso. There are peculiar writing abnormalities large, unequal letters, irregular underlining. This is the classical type of tremor seen in Cerebellar disorders and at such it is also called cerebellar tremor. Cerebellar damage can also produce a "wing-beating" type of tremor called rubral or Holmes' tremor which is actually a combination of rest, action, and postural tremors. *Titubation* is tremor of the head and neck (repeated nodding) is also of cerebellar origin.

10.27 Nystagmus

Nystagmus is a condition of involuntary eye movement. It has been called 'dancing eyes' because of its involuntary nature. It may be congenital like in Sickle cell disease and usually results in reduced or limited vision. The triad of scanning speech, nystagmus and intention tremor is referred to as Charcot's triad (indicative of cerebellar disease).

Memory Impairment

Recently, the cerebellum is being thought to have a part in cognition. Hence patients with cerebellar disorder may exhibit a constellation of subtle to overt cognitive symptoms. Procedural memory loss is one of the cognitive deficits noted.

10.28 Arnold Chiari malformation

This is a congenital malformation that results in downward displacement of the cerebellar tonsil through the foramen magnum. It is a cause of obstructive hydrocephalous.

References

1. Epstein RJ. Medicine for examinations 4th Ed Canada 2006
2. Gates P. The Rule of 4s of the brainstem; a simplified method for understanding brainstem anatomy and brainstem vascular lesions for the non-neurologist Int Med J 2005; 35: 263-266
3. Harold Ellis: Clinical Anatomy 11th Ed Oxford 2006
4. https://en.wikipedia.org/wiki/Reticular_formation
5. Kasper DL, Fauci A S, Hauser S L, Longo D L, Jameson J L, Loscalzo J: Harrison's Principles of Internal Medicine; 19th Ed New York 2015
6. Ropper AH, Brown R H: Adams and Victor' Principles of Neurology 8th Ed New York 2005
7. Swash M, Glynn M: Hutchinson Clinical Methods 22nd Ed Edinburgh 2007
8. Walker HK, Hall WD, Hurst JW; Clinical Methods, The History, Physical, and Laboratory Examinations 3rd Ed Boston 1990

CHAPTER 11
LESIONS OF THE SPINAL CORD

11.0 INTRODUCTION

The hallmark of a spinal cord lesion is the presence of a horizontally defined level below which sensory, motor, and autonomic functions are impaired. During the history taking, the patients will usually delineate this level at which there is weakness, heaviness or numbness below the line on their own. This level is further defined during the sensory examination (pain, temperature or fine touch) where the site of impairment is noted. All the sensory tracts are ascending. The spinothalamic tracts carrying pain, temperature, and fine touch cross over two or three segments after their origin from the sensory receptors. The posterior columns which convey joint position sense and vibration however do not cross over till they get to the medulla where they cross over. There are also features of autonomic disturbances like absence of sweating, bladder, bowel, and sexual dysfunction. Bowel and bladder dysfunction may be *too tight* (urinary retention and constipation) or *too lax* (urinary and faecal incontinence)

In addition, segmental signs caused by disturbed motor and sensory innervations can also localize the uppermost level of a spinal cord lesion. There is also a band of altered sensation (hyperalgesia or hyperpathia) at the upper end of the sensory disturbance. The features of lower motor neurone lesions will be noted at this level. Below the lesion however, there are features of upper motor neurone lesions (hypertonia, hyperreflexia and exaggerated tendon reflexes). However, in some cases, the features of upper motor neurones are not seen in spinal cord lesions. Such persons have features of lower motor neurone lesions. This is referred to as spinal shock. This state of "spinal shock" may last for several days, rarely for weeks. It may be mistaken for extensive damage to the anterior horn cells over many segments of the cord or for an acute polyneuropathy.

The aetiology of spinal cord lesions is classified as shown in Fig 12.

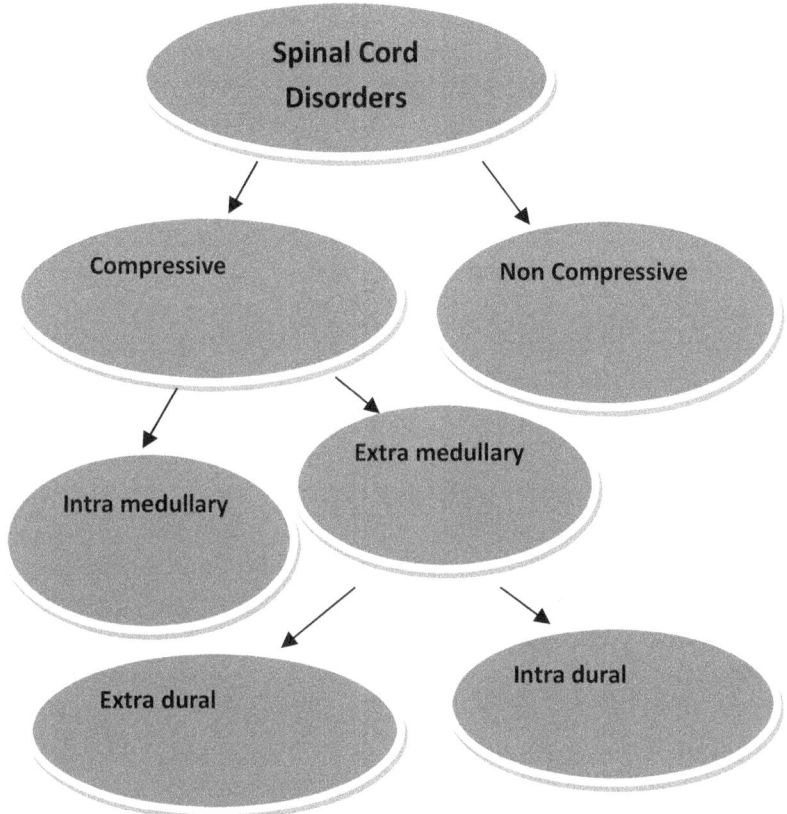

Fig 12: Classification of Lesions in the Spinal Cord

11.10 Levels of lesions

It is important to recognize the horizontal level of the lesion as well as the pattern of the lesion as any of the possible causes can occur at any level.

11.11 Cervical Cord Lesions

Upper Cervical Cord
Lesions of the upper cervical cord lesions classically cause weakness of all the four limbs (quadriparesis or quadriplegia depending on the severity). High cervical cord lesions are frequently life threatening, because of the involvement of C3 to C5. This leads to weakness of the respiratory muscles and paralysis of the diaphragm (C4) with resultant respiratory collapse. In fact, extensive lesions near the medulla are fatal because of the affectation of the vasomotor centres.

Lower cervical cord
Lesions of the lower cervical cord are not fatal. In C5-C6 lesions, there is weakness of the biceps muscle. Further examination will reveal an inverse supinator jerk in which the full supinator jerk is not seen, instead only a brisk flexion of the fingers (C7) will occur. There will be absence of the other components of the supinator jerk which include the biceps jerk (C5, 6), and the supination and flexion components. The author thinks that the more appropriate name should be incomplete Supinator jerk.

In lesions of C7, there is weakness of the extensor muscles of the in middle finger, wrist and triceps whereas C8 lesions cause weakness of the flexors of the finger and wrist.
Horner's syndrome occurs as a result of compression of the cervical sympathetic chain. The features are miosis, ptosis, and facial hypohidrosis. Horner's syndrome may accompany a cervical cord lesion at any level and its presence localises the lesion to the cervical cord and occasionally brain stem depending on other deficits. *Cervical lesions are localized by the muscle weakness not usually the sensory level.*

11.12 Thoracic Cord Lesions
Thoracic lesions classically cause weakness of the lower limbs (paraparesis or paraplegia depending of the severity). Other accompanying features in thoracic cord lesions are numbness (sensory) and disturbances of bladder and bowel function (autonomic). Lesions at T9-T10 also paralyze the lower abdominal

muscles. This is observed as the upward movement of the umbilicus when the abdominal wall contracts (Beevor's sign). Weakness of the upper abdominal muscles will cause the umbilicus to move down on an attempt to rise from the bed. The level of lesions of the thoracic cord is *best localized by the sensory level* on the trunk and, if present, by the site of midline back pain or swelling (gibbus). Note the following useful landmarks.

Male nipple--T4
Xiphisternum--T6
Umblicus--T10
Symphysis Pubis ---T12
 The female nipple is variable.

11.13 Lumbar Cord Lesions
The spinal cord ends somewhere between the first lumbar vertebra (L1) and second lumbar vertebra (L2) as shown in Fig 2. *Consequently, there is no cord in the lumbar and sacral segments of the spine*. Bilateral weakness of the lower limbs (paraparesis, paraplegia) therefore with features suggestive of spinal cord lesion localises the lesion to *above L1*. The common practice of lumbosacral X-Ray or MRI in a patient with paraparesis is inappropriate. The correct site to be investigated should be the thoracic spine.

In lesions at the L2-L4 vertebral levels, there is paralysis flexion and adduction of the thigh with associated weakness leg extension at the knee. The plantar reflex will be flexor.
In lesions at L5-S1 scope of involvement is less with a paralysis of movements of the foot and ankle. There is associated weakness of flexion at the knee, and extension of the thigh. The ankle jerks (S1) are decreased or absent.

11.14 Sacral Cord/Conus Medullaris
 The conusmedullaris syndrome is made up of bilateral saddle anaesthesia (S3-S5 nerve rots). The saddle area corresponds to the concentric rings around the anus (the area used to sit astride like on the saddle of a horse). The sensory impairment in the saddle area is

shown by the different feel of the tissue after defecation. Other features are prominent bladder (urinary retention or incontinence with lax anal tone), bowel dysfunction (constipation or faecal incontinence) and impotence. In some cases, the stools are like pellets. The bulbocavernosus (S2-S4) and anal (S4-S5) reflexes are absent. Note that, muscle strength is largely preserved.

11.15 Cauda Equina lesions
The nerve roots derived from the lower cord form the cauda equina; hence the lesions are characterized by low back and radicular pain. There is associated asymmetric leg weakness and sensory loss, variable areflexia in the lower extremities ('lower motor neurone lesion). In contrast to the conus medullaris lesions, there is relative sparing of bowel and bladder function. Mass lesions in the lower spinal canal often produce a mixed clinical picture with elements of both cauda equina and conus medullaris syndromes

11.20 Patterns of Spinal Cord Disease
The unique arrangement of the major ascending and descending pathways of the spinal cord causes diverse presentations of spinal cord lesions that are easily recognizable. In the spinal cord, the posterior columns and the spinocerebellar and pyramidal tracts are situated on the side of the body they innervate: seeing that the pyramidal tracts had already decussated in the medulla. However, the spinothalamic tract transmitting pain and temperature sensations contralateral to the side they supply: considering they had crossed over two or three segments after their origin.

11.21 Complete transverse cord lesion
This is the simplest pattern to recognize. It presents with radicular pains (band like, girdle like) across the segment. All the functions (motor, sensory and autonomic) below the level of the lesion are impaired or lost including fine touch. There may be hyperaesthesia or parasthesia at the upper level of the lesion. In the cervical cord, the pains radiate to the arms. Common causes are transverse myelitis and trauma. In the thoracic cord, the pain remains circumferential to the chest or abdomen while in the lower thoracic or upper lumbar, the pain radiates to the lower limbs (lancinating).

The impairment or loss of fine touch usually indicates a complete transverse lesion. This is because fine touch runs in both the spinothalamic and posterior columns. In a lesion of one of the tracts, the other compensates hence fine touch will remain intact.

11.22 Brown-Sequard Hemicord Syndrome
There is a lesion of one side of the cord (hemi section of the spinal cord). There is affectation of the descending corticospinal tract at the same side of the lesion (ipsilateral weakness). There is also affectation of the posterior column which ascends without crossing on the same side of the lesion (ipsilateral loss of joint position sense and vibration). In contrast, the affectation of the spinothalamic tract (which had crossed over lower down) will be reflected on the opposite side (contralateral loss of pain and temperature).Segmental signs, such as radicular pain, muscle atrophy, or loss of a deep tendon reflex, are unilateral. Partial forms are more common than the fully developed syndrome.

11.23 Central Cord Syndrome
The central cord syndrome syndrome results from selective damage to the grey matter nerve cells and crossing spinothalamic tracts surrounding the central canal. Central cord syndromes are classically seen in the cervical cord where they produce a characteristic. There is noticeable arm weakness out of proportion to leg weakness. This disproportion results from the fact that within the pyramidal tract, the fibres innervating the upper limbs lie inner while those carrying the lower limbs are outer. Hence, a central lesion will affect the inner fibres earlier with more severity than the outer fibres. The sensory loss is termed "suspended dissociated anaesthesia". The term 'dissociated' signifies the loss of pain and temperature sensations in contrast to preservation of light touch, joint position, and vibration sense. This dissociation is because of the crossing over by the spinothalamic tracts in the middle, hence their affectation by a central lesion. The posterior columns (conveying part of fine touch, joint position sense and vibration) however do not cross over and are far away from the centre of the cord (the site of the lesion). In addition the sensory abnormalities are 'Suspended'over the shoulders, lower neck, and upper trunk (cape distribution). This is because the fibres of the

spinothalamic tracts carrying pain and temperature sensations from the lower limbs crossed over lower down and thereafter continue in the lateral aspect of the cord. The abdomen and lower limbs are therefore spared.

11.24 Anterior Spinal Artery Syndrome/Anterior 2/3rd Syndrome

There is a *single* anterior spinal artery which supplies the anterior two thirds of the spinal cord. Contained in this anterior 2/3rds are the corticospinal tracts on both sides and the spinothalamic tracts. A vascular lesion of this single artery either haemorrhage or infarct will result in bilateral tissue destruction that spares the posterior columns. All spinal cord functions; motor, sensory, and autonomic are lost below the level of the lesion. There is however the preservation of the vibration and position sensation (the posterior column is within the posterior 1/3rd supplied by the posterior spinal arteries).

11.25 Foramen Magnum Syndrome

The spinal cord passes through the foramen magnum as it exits the cranial cavity. It transmits the medulla oblongata and its membranes, the vertebral arteries, the anterior and posterior spinal arteries and the tectorial membranes. The spinal part of the accessory nerve also passes through the foramen magnum into the skull. Lesions in this area interrupt the decussating pyramidal tract fibers destined for the legs. This results in weakness of the legs (*crural paresis*).

Compressive lesions near the foramen magnum may produce the *"around the clock"* pattern of weakness. This is made up of weakness of the ipsilateral shoulder and arm followed by weakness of the ipsilateral leg, then the contralateral leg, and finally the contralateral arm. There is typically sub occipital pain spreading to the neck and shoulders with associated neck stiffness.

11.26 Intramedullary and Extramedullary Syndromes

Spinal cord lesions are classified into intramedullary and extramedullary lesions as shown in Fig 12.

Intramedullary lesions originate within the substance of the cord. Extramedullary lesions on the other hand originate from outside the spinal cord. Extramedullary lesions compress the spinal cord or its vascular supply.

Table 1
Differences between intra and Extramedullary lesions

	Features	Intramedullary	Extra Medullary
1	Pain	Poorly localized burning pain	Prominent radicular (girdle like) pain
2	Weakness	Weakness may precede pain	Pain precedes weakness by weeks or months
3	Sacral Sensation	Perineal and Sacral sparing	Early sacral sensory loss
4	Spasticity	Spasticity is usually late	Spasticity is early
5	Sphincters	Sphincters are intact	Sphincteric disturbance usually incontinence

The differentiating features as shown in Table 1 are only relative and serve as clinical guides. Extramedullary lesions are further divided into Extradural lesions and intradural lesions

Extradural and Intradural
Extradural masses present with pains preceding the weakness over weeks. This is the typical presentation of tuberculosis of the spine (Potts Disease). Acute abscesses present earlier. Most other lesions that cause extradural cord compression are malignant like secondaries from other sites. An uncommon cause of extradural compression in the tropics is ova of schistosoma and the latter benign (neurofibroma being a common cause). Consequently, a long duration of symptoms favors an intradural origin.

11.27 Compressive and Non Compressive Spinal cord lesions

Compressive cord lesions include the following;
Vascular: Aneurysms, AVMs, Anterior spinal artery haemorrhage
Infectious causes: Staphylococcal epidural abscess, Spine TB (Potts disease), ova of Schistosoma
Cystic disease: Syringomyelia, Arachnoid cysts
Tumours: Benign like Neuroma, Fibroma, Neurofibroma, Shwanoma, Meningoma, and Lipoma
Malignant: Astrocytoma, Multiple Myeloma and Secondaries from Prostate, Breast, Lungs, Bladder, Colon etc
Traumatic causes; vertebral fracture, disc herniation, epidural haemorrhage
Spine abnormalities; Scoliosis, kyphosis
Degenerative causes; Spondylosis, Spondylolisthesis

Non Compressive lesions include the following:
Infectious: Transverse myelitis from a variety of organisms
Viral: Epstein Barr virus, Coxsackie virus, HIV, Varicella Zoster virus, Herpes Simplex virus, Adenoviruses, enteroviruses, HTLV 1 and 11
Bacteria; Staph Aureus, Streptococci,
Spirochetes; Syphilis, Lyme disease
Fungi; Cryptococcus, Aspergillosis
Demyelinating disease: Multiple sclerosis, Neuromyelitis optica
Vascular: Spinal artery infarct, Vasculitides like PAN, SLE
Toxins; Lathyrism, konzo, Zinc, Arsenic etc
Degenerative disorders: Primary Lateral Sclerosis, Familial Spastic Paraparesis, Spinocerebellar Ataxia, Freidrich's Ataxia
Metabolic; Vitamin deficiencies like Sub acute combined degeneration of the cord (SACD) from Vitamin B_{12} Def, Vitamin E Def, Folic acid deficiency, Chronic Kidney Disease, Hepatic failure
Para neoplastic causes; lymphoma and several carcinomas

References
1. Baliga R R: 250 short cases in clinical Medicine 3rd Ed Saunders 2001.
2. Ekeh Bertha C; Clinical Neurology made Easy 1st Ed USA 2018
3. Epstein RJ. Medicine for examinations 4th Ed Canada 2006
4. Kasper DL, Fauci A S, Hauser S L, Longo D L, Jameson J L, Loscalzo J: Harrison's Principles of Internal Medicine; 19th Ed New York 2015
5. Lindsay K W. Bone I: Neurology and Neurosurgery Illustrated 4th Ed Edinburgh 2005
6. Ropper AH, Brown R H: Adams and Victor' Principles of Neurology 8th Ed New York 2005
7. Swash M, Glynn M: Hutchinson Clinical Methods 22nd Ed Edinburgh 2007
8. University of Texas: Neuroscience online, an electronic textbook for NeuroSciences

CHAPTER 12

LESIONS OF THE PERIPHERAL NERVES

12.0 Introduction

The peripheral nervous system as earlier discussed refers to parts of the nervous system outside the brain and spinal cord. It comprises the cranial nerves as well as the spinal nerves all through their course. The anterior horn cells are included because they are part of the motor unit. Sensory nerves receive sensation, such as temperature, pain, vibration or touch, from the skin. In sensory neuropathies, the patients have various complaints of sensory disturbances as described below.

Motor nerves control the muscle movement. In motor neuropathies, there is weakness of the particular muscles or group

Autonomic functions include control of respiration, regulation of the cardiac (the cardiac control center) and vasomotor activity (the vasomotor center). Others are certain reflex actions such as coughing, sneezing, swallowing and vomiting. Every organ in the body has a sympathetic and parasympathetic nerve supply with one division generating the opposite effect to the other. Dysfunction of the autonomic nervous system leads to poor control of many systems such as blood pressure, heart rate, digestion and sphincter control.

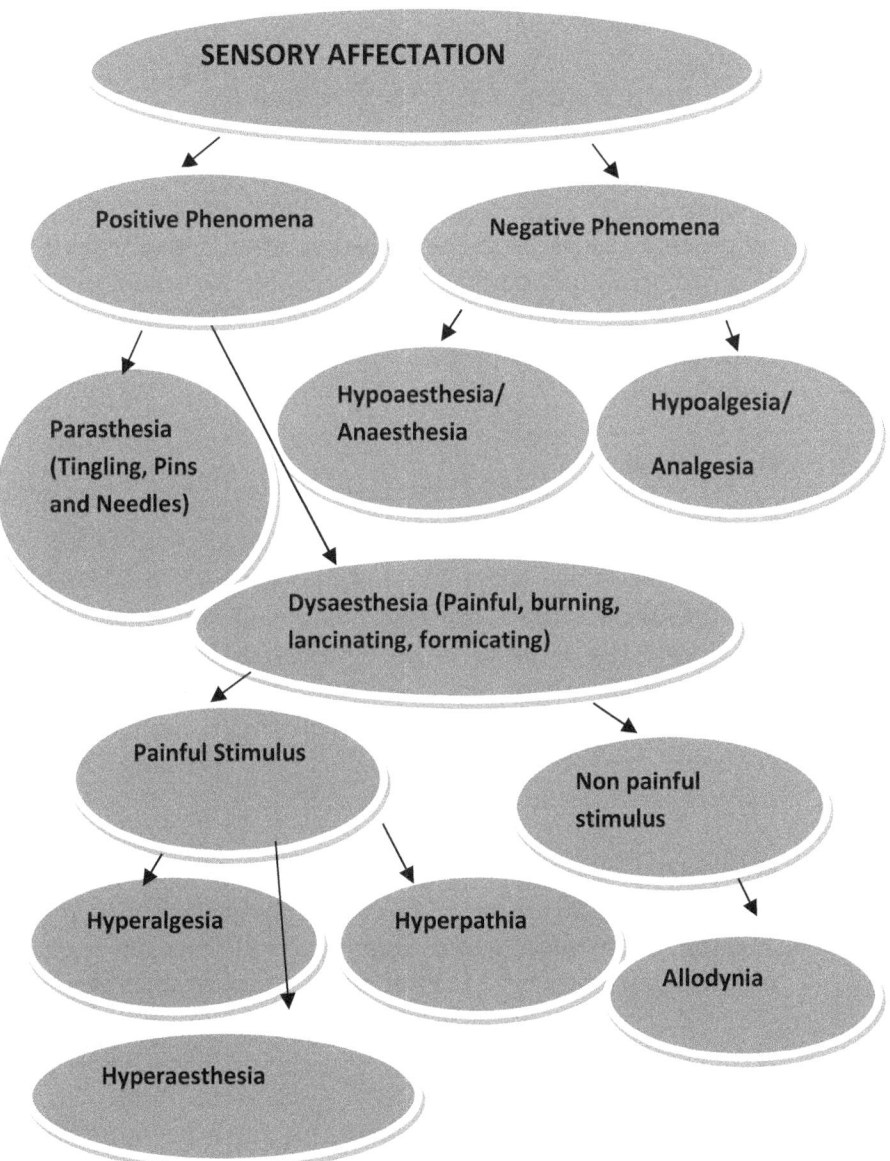

Fig 13: Classification of Sensory symptoms

12.10 Sensory Neuropathy; Disturbances in sensory nerves are classified as shown in Fig 13. They may present with positive or negative phenomenon.

12.11 Positive symptoms present as follows:

Parasthesia This refers to an abnormal sensation that is often described as tingling or numbness, skin crawling, or itching. The sensation is usually felt in the hands, arms, legs, or feet, but can also occur in other parts of the body. *The sensation is abnormal, but it is not unpleasant or painful.* Classically, the person complains of pin and needles sensation or a feeling of walking on cotton wool.

Dysaesthesia

This is defined as an unpleasant, abnormal sense of touch. It often presents as pain but may also present as an inappropriate, uncomfortable sensations. This unpleasant abnormal sensation is not necessarily painful. It includes hyperalgesia, hyperaesthesia and allodynia. There are complaints of burning or excruciating pains. Others are lancinating, burning, shooting, freezing, cramping and formicating (feeling of crawling ants). These sensations are usually worse in the night.

Hyperaesthesia
In hyperaesthesia, there is an increased sensitivity to stimulation including hyperalgesia and allodynia. It involves an abnormal increase in sensitivity to stimuli of the sensory modalities.

Hyperalgesia

In hyperalgesia there is an increased response to a normally painful stimulus (only the pain modality) e.g. a pinprick feels like a knife stab. The stimulus is painful but the sensitivity to pains is markedly exaggerated.

Allodynia

In allodynia, there is pain resulting from a stimulus that will not usually provoke pain e.g. a finger touch or an item of clothing causes pain. This is because of an implicit change in the sensory quality of stimulus. It is different from hyperalgesia where the stimulus is painful but the response is exaggerated.

Hyperpathia

Hyperpathia is derived from two words (*hyper* above and *pathia* suffering i.e. above or too much suffering) It is actually a type of hyperalgesia. In hyperpathia, there is also exaggerated response to a noiceptive stimulus or even no stimulus at all. The abnormal pain response is usually explosive, expanded radiation and of extreme severity to an often repetitive stimulus applied to an area of decreased sensitivity. In essence, the pain continues even when the stimulus is removed.

12.12 Negative Symptoms

Anaesthesia/Hypoaesthesia

Anaesthesia means "loss of sensation". There is loss of all the sensory modalities. The person will usually complain of numbness of the limb or the affected part of the body. They are vulnerable to injuries because of the absence of sensation. Pain and temperature sensations are protective and alert therefore the person to withdraw from the stimulus. This is common in Diabetic neuropathies.

Analgesia /Hypoalgesia

This is the absence or reduction of pain sensation only. Other sensory modalities are intact. The person may complain of numbness. The person is also vulnerable to injuries because of the loss of pain sensation which is protective.

12.20 Motor neuropathy

The dysfunction of the motor neurones leads to weakness of muscles or paralysis. Sensory neuron dysfunction results in abnormal or lost sensation. Some disorders are progressive and fatal.

A motor unit is made up of an anterior horn cell, its motor axon, the innervated muscle fibers as well as the connection between them (neuromuscular junction). The anterior horn cells are located in the grey matter of the spinal cord and thus are technically part of the CNS. Nerve fibers outside the spinal cord join to form roots. The anterior (ventral) roots are the motor nerve roots while the posterior (dorsal) are the sensory nerve roots. These ventral and dorsal roots unite to form a spinal nerve. All the spinal nerve pairs have dorsal and ventral roots except the first cervical nerve (C1) which has no sensory root. Features associated with lesions of the peripheral nerves are muscle weakness, twitching, paralysis and loss of coordination. Others are lack of coordination and falling.

Motor neuropathies show the features of lower motor neurone lesions. These are the weakness of muscles which is limited to the muscle, groups of muscles or a root innervated pattern. The muscles will be wasted. Other features are hypotonia or atonia in the limb. Other features are diminished or absent tendon reflexes (hyporeflexia or areflexia). Muscle wasting, fasciculations and fibrillations are typically signs of end-stage muscle denervation and are seen over a longer time period. Fasciculations are elicited manually while fibrillations are elicited electrically. One defining feature is the segmentation of symptoms; *only muscles innervated by the damaged nerves will be symptomatic* e.g. foot drop after a common peroneal nerve injury.

12.30 Autonomic Neuropathy

Every organ in the body has both sympathetic and sympathetic systems. Autonomic lesions therefore affect every organ. Usually there are both symptoms of both sympathetic and parasympathetic dysfunction and they are so many. Occasionally the presentation is that of generalized dysautonomia. Observable sites of autonomic dysfunction on clinical evaluation include the following;

Face
Classical features seen on the face are flushing, pallor and anhidrosis (absence of sweating).

Vision
There may be blurring then graying of vision, blacking out, tunnel vision, sensitivity to light, difficulty with focusing, reduced lacrimation, and loss of pupillary size over time (which is often correlated with loss of visual symptoms). There may be an associated Horner's syndrome. In some cases there is xerostomia and xerophthalmia (dry mouth and dry eyes).

Cardiovascular system
In autonomic dysfunction, certain changes occur in the blood pressure on standing up leading to palpitations, pre-syncope with light-headedness and visual blurring. *Orthostatic hypotension* is one of the examination findings. In orthostatic hypotension, there is a reduction of systolic blood pressure by more than 20 mm Hg or reduction of diastolic blood pressure by more than 10mmHg in the erect position. Postural tachycardia syndrome is present if tachycardia response is excessive (>30 beats/min increase from baseline).

Gastrointestinal tract
Gastrointestinal symptoms are many. Common symptoms are constipation, nocturnal diarrhea and bowel incontinence. Others include gastroparesis which may cause food stasis and subsequent vomiting. There may also be pre-syncope with micturition, and defecation.

Renal
Urinary tract features include nocturia, bladder urgency, bladder frequency, enuresis, incomplete bladder voiding, urinary retention, and urinary incontinence. Examination may reveal a distended bladder.

Sexual dysfunction
This is common in autonomic dysfunction. This may be impotence, loss of ejaculation, and retrograde ejaculation in men; inability to achieve orgasm or nonspecific sexual dysfunction in both sexes.

Sweating abnormalities
There may be reduced or absence of sweating (anhidrosis or hypohidrosis). Some may have excessive sweating (hyperhidrosis), and sweating after a meal (gustatory sweating).

Temperature regulation
There is occurrence of hypothermia. This results from loss of shivering and inability to vasoconstrict to prevent heat loss in addition to hyperpyrexia.

In neuropathy there may be the affectation of one nerve (mononeuropathy). There may also be the affectation of two or more nerves in different areas (multiple mononeuropathy). In some cases, many nerves (polyneuropathy) are affected. Carpal tunnel syndrome is a classical example of mononeuropathy. The commonest type of neuropathy is the polyneuropathy.

12.40 Cranial Nerve Lesions
Diseases of the cranial nerves are usually seen in the head since the cranial nerves carry somatosensory information to the head and neck.

Olfactory lesion
In olfactory nerve lesions, there is the impaired perception and or identification of smell (anosmia). An important sign in the diagnosis of frontal lobe tumours is the presence of unilateral

anosmia. Lesions of the uncus may cause a characteristic type of seizures referred to as 'uncinate' seizures. The features are olfactory hallucinations with associated impairment of consciousness as well as involuntary chewing movements.

Optic nerve lesion

Features of optic nerve lesions are as follows;

Ptosis (drooping of the eyelids) results from paralysis of either of or two of the muscles that open the eyelid: Muller's muscle or the levator palpebrae superioris. Thus ptosis is a feature of both optic and occulomotor nerve palsies. *In optic nerve palsy, the eye with ptosis has a smaller pupil and the eye movements are full while in occulomotor nerve palsy, the eye with the ptosis has a larger or a normal pupil.*

Blindness

Lesions of the retina or optic nerve result in ipsilateral blindness in the affected segment. Monocular blindness is the visual loss in one eye. It may appear as blindness, dimming, fogging or blurring. It usually indicates an ocular lesion. This may occur in seconds or minutes in cases of amaurosis fugax: a type of transient ischaemic attack. Binocular blindness however is a feature of a cerebral lesion: cortical blindness (Anton syndrome).

Hemianopia

Hemianopia (*hemi* half, *anopia* without vision) is blindness over one half of the visual field. Lesions of the occipital lobe result in contralateral *homonymous hemianopia* (loss of vision on the same side of both eyes).

Similarly, lesions of the optic chiasma (e.g. from an expanding pituitary tumour) will give rise to a *bitemporal hemianopia*, i.e. there will be a loss of vision in both temporal eye-fields.

Light –Near Dissociation

Having tested the light reflex, there is usually no need to check the near response (Accommodation) if the pupils respond briskly to light, because an isolated loss of constriction (meiosis) to accommodation does not occur. However, it is important to test the near response if the light response is poor or absent. Positive response of the pupil to accommodation in the absence of brisk response to light (*Light-Near dissociation*) is seen to occur rarely in the following conditions; Argyll Robertson pupil, Parinaud's syndrome and Adie Tonic Pupil (Holmes-Adie Syndrome). The lesion responsible for the *Argyll Robertson pupil* is thought to be in the vicinity of the pretectal area.

Occulomotor nerve lesion
Ptosis
Features of occulomotor nerve palsy include ptosis (drooping of the eyelids) due to paralysis of the levator palpebrae superioris. The eye with the ptosis has a larger or normal size pupil. Compressive brain lesions are common causes of unilateral ptosis. Another defining feature is a *divergent squint*. This occurs as a result of the unopposed action of the superior oblique and lateral rectus muscles. The person will also notice double vision Examination reveals dilatation of pupil and the loss of accommodation-light convergence.

Lesions of the occulomotor nucleus in the brain stem have been described above in chapter 9.

Trochlear nerve lesion
There is also a squint. The eye is 'down and out'.

Trigeminal nerve lesion

Section of the whole trigeminal nerve results in unilateral anaesthesia of the face, the auricle and the anterior part of the scalp. The mucous membranes of the nose, mouth and anterior two-thirds of the tongue are also involved. In addition, there is associated paralysis and wasting of the muscles of mastication. Lesions of separate divisions give rise to corresponding sensory and motor deficits in the area of distribution of the affected nerve. The main motor deficit is inability to chew because of the weakness of the masseter muscles. Trigeminal neuralgia may affect any one or more of the three divisions, giving rise to the characteristic pain over the appropriate area. Pain is frequently referred from one segment to another.

Abducens nerve lesion
A lesion of the abducens nerve also causes a squint. Abducens nucleus can be involved in brain stem lesions as described in chapter 9.

Gradenigo's syndrome
Lesions at the petrous apex like mastoiditis can produce deafness, pain, and ipsilateral abducens palsy.

Cavernous sinus syndrome
The cavernous sinus contains the Occulomotor (3rd), Trochlear (4th), Trigeminal (5th) and Abducens (6th) nerves. These nerves are paralysed in cavernous sinus thrombosis. Abducens nerve palsy is the commonest nerve palsy. There is usually involvement of the sensory branches of the Ophthalmic and Maxillary the 5th nerve. Unilateral or bilateral abducens palsy is a classic sign of raised intracranial pressure. The clinical diagnosis can be made on fundoscopy where papilloedema is observed. The mechanism is still debated but probably is related to rostral-caudal displacement of the brainstem.

Facial nerve lesion
All the muscles of facial expression including taste sensation from the anterior two-thirds of the tongue are supplied by the facial nerve. A lesion of the facial nerve causes weakness of the muscles of facial expression. There is associated loss of taste over the anterior two-thirds of the tongue. Other features are hyperacusis due to the paralysis of the stapedius which dampens the noise. Other symptoms are deafness, tinnitus or dizziness. It is important to distinguish between lesions above the nucleus (upper motor neurone lesions) and the lesions involving the nucleus and below the nucleus (lower motor neurone lesions). Lower motor neurone lesions result in complete paralysis of one side of the face while in upper motor neurone lesions; there is no involvement of the muscles above the palpebral fissures. This is because the portion of the facial nucleus supplying these muscles receives fibres from both cerebral hemispheres. The commonest cause of lower motor neurone lesion of the facial nerve is Bell's palsy.

Vestibulocochlear nerve lesion

Lesions of the cochlear division result in deafness which may, or may not, be accompanied by tinnitus. There may be dysacusis. Apart from injury to the cochlear nerve itself, unilateral lesions of the auditory pathway do not greatly affect auditory acuity because of the bilaterality of the auditory projections. Temporal lobe tumours may give rise to auditory hallucinations if they encroach upon the auditory (superior temporal) gyrus.
Lesions of the vestibulocerebellar pathway or the vestibular division of the labyrinth pathway result in vertigo. There is associated instability, loss of balance and vomiting.

Glossopharyngeal nerve lesion
Taste and swallowing
A lesion of the glossopharyngeal nerve results in sensory loss in the pharynx, loss of taste over the posterior one third of the tongue. There is associated pharyngeal weakness leading to hoarseness and difficulty in swallowing. Such lesions however are so often associated involvement of the Vagus or its nuclei.

Vagus nerve lesion
Lesions of the Vagus and glossopharyngeal nerves usually occur together as earlier mentioned. There is difficulty in swallowing (Dysphagia) and difficulty in phonation (Dysphonia). In addition, the gag reflex is also lost. The voice is hoarse and slightly nasal. There may also be regurgitation of liquids through the nose occurs during swallowing. In unilateral paralysis, the uvula deviates to the normal side when the patient says 'Ah'.

Accessory nerve lesion
The person will be unable to shrug. There may be associated weakness of the neck muscles.

Hypoglossal nerve lesion

Lesions of the hypoglossal nerve, or lesions involving its nucleus, result in an ipsilateral paralysis and wasting of the muscles of the tongue. This is detected clinically by deviation of the protruded tongue to the affected side. Supranuclear paralysis (due to an upper motor neurone lesion involving the corticobulbar pathways) leads to paresis but not atrophy of the muscles of the contralateral side.

12.50 Multiple cranial nerve palsies

Certain disorders may affect several cranial nerves. It is therefore pertinent to determine whether the lesion lies within the brainstem or outside it. In lesions within the brainstem, there is early involvement of the long tracts (sensory and motor) with the cranial nerve deficits. Lesions that are superficial to the brainstem are characterized by involvement of adjacent cranial nerves. These generally occur one after the other. The features of the involvement of the long tracts appear late. Brain stem lesions also cause a characteristic crossed paralysis in which the cranial nerve signs are on one side of the body and the tract signs are on the opposite side.
Multiple cranial nerve palsies therefore form a number of distinctive syndromes.

The cavernous sinus syndrome is a distinctive syndrome. It often presents as orbital or swelling, facial pain and fever. There are multiple cranial nerve palsies including the 3rd, 4th, and 6th cranial nerves. In addition there is an associated trigeminal neuropathy affecting the ophthalmic (V1) and occasionally the maxillary (V2) divisions. Cavernous sinus thrombosis, often secondary to infection from orbital cellulitis (frequently *Staphylococcus aureus*), a cutaneous source on the face, or sinusitis (especially with mucormycosis in diabetic patients), is commonest cause. The two cavernous sinuses directly communicate via intercavernous channels; thus, involvement on one side may extend to become bilateral. Occasionally, there may be an idiopathic form of multiple cranial nerve palsies of the face. This may be unilateral or bilateral. The clinical features are similar to features of the Tolosa-Hunt syndrome. The pathology seems to be idiopathic inflammation of the dura mater. The inflammation may be seen on MRI. The syndrome is usually responsive to glucocorticoids.

12.60 Plexopathies

Plexopathies involve the specific network (plexus) of nerves. It can involve
The Brachial plexus
The Lumbar plexus
The Sacral plexus

Brachial plexopathy
All the muscles of the shoulder girdle and upper extremities are supplied by the brachial plexus. Lesions of the brachial plexus cause weakness, sensory loss, and loss of tendon reflexes in these areas.

Lumbar plexopathy
Lesions of the lumbar plexus produce weakness, sensory loss, and reflex changes in the distribution of spinal segments L1-L4, resulting in weakness and sensory loss in obturator- and femoral-innervated territories.

Sacral plexopathy
Lesions of the sacral plexus cause the same abnormalities in segments L5-S3, causing weakness and sensory loss in the gluteal (motor only), peroneal and tibial nerve territories.

References

1. Ekeh Bertha C; Clinical Neurology made Easy 1st Ed USA 2018
2. Epstein RJ. Medicine for examinations 4th Ed Canada 2006
3. Harold Ellis: Clinical Anatomy 11th Ed Oxford 2006
4. Kasper DL, Fauci A S, Hauser S L, Longo D L, Jameson J L, Loscalzo J: Harrison's Principles of Internal Medicine; 19th Ed New York 2015
5. Lindsay K W. Bone I: Neurology and Neurosurgery Illustrated 4th Ed Edinburgh 2005
6. Ropper AH, Brown R H: Adams and Victor' Principles of Neurology 8th Ed New York 2005
7. Swash M, Glynn M: Hutchinson Clinical Methods 22nd Ed Edinburgh 2007
8. University of Texas: Neuroscience online, an electronic textbook for NeuroSciences

CHAPTER 13

LESIONS OF THE NEURO MUSCULAR JUNCTION AND MUSCLES

13.10 Lesions of The Neuromuscular Junction

The cardinal features are neuromuscular junction disorders are *weakness* and *fatigability* of muscles.

13.11 Weakness

Muscle weakness is the classical feature of neuromuscular junction disorders (classically Myasthenia gravis). The weakness is usually generalized and intermittent usually resolving after sleep or rest.

Cranial muscles involvement

Cranial muscles involvement
The cranial muscles are affected early in myasthenia gravis. This is characteristic. Muscles of the eyelids and the extraocular muscles are often the earliest muscles involved. Hence ptosis (drooping) of the eyelids and diplopia (double vision) are usually the first complaints in as much as 50% of cases. *In fact the occurrence of bilateral drooping of the eyelids (ptosis) is almost pathognomonic for Myasthenia Gravis.* In some cases weakness the muscles of the face, jaws, neck and throat is the initial symptoms ; though this is not very often.

The person's smile becomes a snarl because of the weakness of the face. Weakness in chewing is most noticeable after prolonged effort, as in chewing meat. The weakness of the tongue and palate causes a mushy timbre to the speech. Thereafter there is difficulty in swallowing with associated regurgitation of food. In some cases there may be aspiration. The initial affectation of the limb muscles is infrequent.

Proximal myopathy

The general muscle weakness typically involves the *proximal muscles* in a symmetric manner (proximal myopathy). The person will complain of difficulty in movements that require the use of the proximal muscles. The proximal muscles of the lower limbs (hamstrings and quadriceps) are the largest and weight bearing joints; weakness of these muscles leads to difficulty is climbing the stair case, rising from a seated position. In severe cases, there is associated frequent falls. Involvement of the upper limbs (weakness of the pectoral girdle) causes difficulty in raising the hands above the head. Chores like fixing a bulb or cleaning the ceiling fan become difficult. The classic gait is *waddling or myopathic gait* (duck like) caused by the weakness of the hip muscles leading to hip drop or dip. Hyperextension of the knee (genu recurvatum or back-kneeing) is characteristic of quadriceps muscle weakness.

13.12 Fatigability
Fatigability is increasing weakness during repeated use or late in the day. There is a characteristic improvement after sleep or rest. In essence, the weakness is intermittent.

Asthenia
Asthenia is a type of fatigue caused by excess tiredness or lack of energy and may be confused with fatigability. Associated symptoms may help differentiate asthenia and pathologic fatigability. In persons with asthenia, there is daytime sleepiness leading to frequent naps. Hence they tend to avoid physical activities. They also have difficulty in concentration. This affects activities like reading. They may also have stress and depression. Thus, asthenia is not a myopathy. Persons with myopathy do not avoid physical activities. They do not feel sleepy in the daytime and as such do not take naps. In addition they do not have stress and depression. Pathologic fatigability also occurs in chronic myopathies. This leads to less accomplished tasks.

13.20 Lesions of Muscles/Myopathies

Muscle diseases also present with weakness. The weakness is also usually proximal and symmetric either involving the arms, legs or both. Most muscle diseases however cause *persistent generalized symmetric proximal weakness* (proximal myopathy) as against neuromuscular junction disorders where the weakness is *intermittent*. More so muscle disorders generally spare the cranial muscles except in few cases like the facio-scapulo-humeral dystrophy and myotonic dystrophy. In few cases, a unique category of muscular dystrophies which cause asymmetric and predominantly *distal weakness* can also be seen in some myopathies (distal myopathies).These distal myopathies cause difficulty in movements that need distal muscles like clenching the fists or pedalling bicycle. The gait abnormality in distal myopathies is the slapping gait or foot drop. It is pertinent to examine what functions are impaired in order to determine the pattern of weakness.

Muscular Dystrophy

Muscular dystrophy is made up of a group of muscle diseases. There are more than 30 diseases in all. These diseases cause muscle weakness and degeneration over time. They primarily affect only muscles but some may have associated affectation of other muscles. The disorders differ in the specific muscles affected, the beginning of the symptoms and the speed of the degeneration. They are caused by gene mutations in the genes involved in building muscle proteins. The disorders may be X-linked recessive, autosomal recessive or autosomal dominant. The most common is Duchenne muscular Dystrophy (DMD) which affects males and begins at the age of 4 years: caused by mutation in the dystrophin gene. Invariably most of the boys with Duchenne are in a wheel chair by the age of 12. Becker muscular dystrophy is a milder form: starts later than Duchenne and progresses slower. Others include facioscapulohumeral muscular dystrophy and myotonic dystrophy. Involvement of the cardio respiratory muscles is life threatening.

Table 2: Distinguishing the Origin of Weakness

SIGN	UMN	LMN	MYOPATHY	PSYCHOGENIC	NMJ
Wasting	None	Severe	Mild	None	None
Fasciculations	None	Present	None	None	None
Tone	Spastic May be reduced in Spinal shock	Flaccid	Normal or Decreased	Variable or Paratonia	Normal or Decreased
Distribution of Weakness	Pyramidal/ Regional	Distal/ Segmental	Proximal	Variable/ inconsistent with daily activities	Proximal
Tendon Reflex	Hperactive or Exaggerated It may be hypoactive in Spinal shock	Hypoactive/ Absent	Normal or Hypoactive	Normal	Normal or Hypoactive
Plantar Response	Exaggerated May be flexor in Spinal shock	Flexor	Flexor	Flexor	Flexor

13.11 Causes of muscle diseases include the following:

Genetic causes
Muscular dystrophy: Duchenne, Becker, Facioscapulohumeral
Acquired Causes
Infections: HIV, Coxsackie A and B, Influenza, Lyme disease, Trichinosis, cystercercosis, Toxoplasmosis
Inflammatory myopathies; Polymyositis, Dermatomyositis, Inclusion body myositis
Neuromuscular junction Disorders: Myasthenia Gravis
Endocrine and Metabolic; Thyroid disorders, Addison's, Cushing's, Parathyroid disease
Medications/Toxins; Statins, Steroids, Colcichine, Alcohol
Electrolyte Abnormalities; Hyper/Hypokalaemic periodic paralysis

13.30 SUMMARY OF SITE OF LESIONS

Cerebral Cortex
a. Presence of cognitive deficits
b. Visual field hemianopias and quadrantanopias
c. Hemisensory Loss
d. Hemiparesis
e. Loss of Olfaction
f. Loss of Consciousness
g. Reappearance of primitive reflexes
h. Focal or generalized seizures

Brainstem
a. Presence of cranial nerve deficits.
b. Internuclear ophthalmoplegia
c. Crossed paralysis.
d. Loss of consciousness

Cerebellum
a. Ataxia
b. Intention tremor
c. Scanning Dysarthria
d. Dysmetria
e. Dysdiadochokinesia
f. Nystagmus

Spinal Cord
a. Deficits (motor and sensory) that fit a dermatomal distribution which start at a specific dermatome and include all the dermatomes below
b. Motor deficits are ipsilateral
c. Sensory deficits may vary depending on the pattern
d. May involve the sphincters

Spinal nerve roots
  a. Deficits restricted to single dermatome that are purely sensory or motor

Peripheral nerves
  a. Non dermatomal deficit that fits distribution of a peripheral nerve
  b. Stocking-glove distribution of deficits
  c. Non dermatomal deficit that involves sensory only or motor only symptoms
  d. Lower motor neurone lesion

Neuromuscular Junction
  a. Intermittent generalized weakness(proximal)
  b. Fatigability
  c. Early cranial muscle involvement

Muscle Disease
  a. Persistent symmetric weakness(Proximal)
  b. Sparing of cranial muscles
  c. Recognized patterns

References

1. Ekeh Bertha C; Clinical Neurology made Easy 1st Ed USA 2018
3. Epstein RJ. Medicine for examinations 4th Ed Canada 2006
4. Harold Ellis: Clinical Anatomy 11th Ed Oxford 2006
5. Kasper DL, Fauci A S, Hauser S L, Longo D L, Jameson J L, Loscalzo J: Harrison's Principles of Internal Medicine; 19th Ed New York 2015
6. Ropper AH, Brown R H: Adams and Victor' Principles of Neurology 8th Ed New York 2005
7. Swash M, Glynn M: Hutchinson Clinical Methods 22nd Ed Edinburgh 2007

CHAPTER 14

MAPPING AND IDENTIFYING THE PATHOLOGY

14.0 Introduction
The issue of localizing the site and level of lesion in the neuraxis has been defined in the previous chapters. The next logical step is mapping out the lesion. This will ascertain not just the location but the pattern and degree of involvement.

14.10 Mapping
The possibilities to be considered are as follows: is the lesion focal, multifocal, diffuse, part of a multi-system or a combination?

Focal lesions
In a focal lesion all the features of the condition can be accounted for by a single, discrete neuroanatomical locus. They are usually the easiest lesions to localize. Focal lesions are usually single infarcts, specific tumours, trauma and mononeuropathies. Some examples are lacunar infarcts that involve the deep penetrating arteries of the cortex. Common symptoms may be sudden inability to speak, deviation of the mouth to one side, sudden loss of sensation or slight weakness of the arm. Specific tumours like a pituitary adenoma compressing the optic chiasma present with headaches and visual field defects. Another common example of a focal neurological lesion is a mononeuropathy like Bell's palsy or carpal tunnel syndrome.

Multifocal process

A multifocal process involves more than one locus. In these conditions, the same pathology affects multiple discrete sites. The lesion affects distinct isolated aspects of the structure while sparing some others. Examples of multifocal processes include multiple infarcts, mononeuritis multiplex and multiple sclerosis. In nononeuritis multiplex, there is involvement of multiple specific nerves (e.g., median, ulnar, and femoral). All nerves will not be involved.

Multiple Sclerosis

The prototype of a multifocal neurological disease is multiple sclerosis (MS). *Multiple sclerosis is an immune-mediated inflammatory disease which attacks myelinated axons. It destroys the myelin and the axon in variable degrees. The attacks of MS may be so diverse and wide apart, such that the symptoms seem unconnected.* *In fact the hallmark of MS is symptomatic episodes that occur months or years apart and affect different anatomic locations.* Some classic MS symptoms are as follows: sensory loss (peripheral nerve involvement), motor features (spinal cord), autonomic feature or features of cerebellar dysfunction. Other common features are visual symptoms include pain, depression some cognitive deficits and constitutional symptoms. Actually, the features may be so diverse and far apart that they are considered as being different pathologies. Moreover the symptoms and severity vary widely amongst different patients. Some people with severe MS may lose the ability to either walk or can only walk with support while others may experience long periods of remission without any new symptoms

Diffuse lesions

In diffuse lesions, there is a widespread dysfunction of a part of the nervous system. Such lesions include encephalopathy due to a variety of metabolic or toxic causes, dementia; numbness and pain in a glove and stocking distribution. This occurs due to diabetic small fiber peripheral neuropathy. One example of a diffuse disease is the distal symmetrical polyneuropathy. In this condition, **all the axons** are involved. The disease affects the distal-most portion. The resultant effect is the classical glove and stocking sensory impairment as well as motor loss. Multifocal and diffuse lesions are always difficult to differentiate from each other. This is because there is involvement of more than one discrete physical location. *The difference is that the lesions remain discrete in a multifocal process (same lesion in different foci sparing some foci), whereas in diffuse, there is a generalized (none is spared) dysfunction.* Noteworthy is the fact that the multifocal processes may eventually progress to a generalized diffuse involvement.

Component of a systemic disease
The final type is that the neurological lesion may be a component of a systemic disease (multisystem) process. This is common in infectious diseases, metabolic disorders, malignancies, connective tissue disorders. Some examples include headache and tremors in thyrotoxicosis, peripheral neuropathies and headaches in Systemic lupus erythemathosus. It may also be a component of a general insult e.g. trauma, encephalitis, anoxia, intoxication or poisoning. In some cases, there may be medically unexplained symptoms.

14.20 Identify the Pathology/Aetiology
It is pertinent to emphasize that the fundamental steps in diagnosis always involve the accurate elicitation of symptoms and signs and their proper interpretation. It is inappropriate to seek the cause of a disease of the nervous system without first ascertaining the parts or structures that are affected. In essence, the anatomic diagnosis takes precedence over the pathologic diagnosis. In cases of doubt, it is wise to examine the patient all over again as it is said that *"a second examination is the most helpful diagnostic test in a difficult neurologic case"*. Discerning the cause of a clinical syndrome (aetiologic diagnosis) requires more knowledge in other aspects. Here the clinician must be conversant with the other clinical details, including the mode of onset, course, and natural history of a many disease entities. These are pertinent on addressing the question "What is the lesion?"

All disorders fall into two broad classifications:
Congenital
Acquired

Congenital
Congenital lesions are pathologies present at birth. Brain development begins shortly after conception and continues throughout the growth of a fetus. The damage of normal brain development of this program, especially when it occurs early in development, can cause structural defects in the brain. Congenital brain defects may be caused by inherited genetic defects, spontaneous mutations within the genes of the embryo, or effects

on the embryo due to the mother's infection, trauma, or drug use. Congenital neurologic pathologies like spina bifida are commonly seen on children. Genetic disorders and in borne errors of metabolism affecting the nervous system also manifest in childhood.

Acquired
The acquired lesions result from brain damage caused by events after birth. Acquired is further reclassified into;
Infectious
Traumatic
Degenerative
Toxic
Metabolic
Deficiency
Inherited
Neoplastic
Inflammatory-immune

The temporal profile of the symptoms is of utmost importance in the clinical evaluation in order to ascertain the pathology. It then follows that the history should be taken in the chronological order of the symptoms. It is important to define the very first symptom to guide the assessment. Some diseases have characteristic features like Tetanus. The typical history is that of a deep contuted wound followed days later by lock jaw and spasms. At such times, there may not be need to follow the stepwise process. In some cases, it is not necessary to carry the clinical analysis beyond the stage of the anatomic diagnosis. This is common in neuropathies like in Bells palsy, carpal tunnel syndrome and in cases of trauma. The aetiology in such cases is usually vascular, trauma, infectious, metabolic or toxic.

14.21 Temporal Profile/Course of the Illness
Determining the precise time of appearance and rate of progression of the symptoms experienced by the patient is paramount. A common error occurs when the patient considers the long standing symptoms supposedly innocuous. Such patients concentrate on giving the history of the more recent dramatic

events. One way of avoiding this is asking 'What was the very first thing you noticed'? It is pertinent to ensure that the history is taking in a chronological order. Hence a two year history of forgetfulness may indicate Alzheimer disease whereas a history of sudden forgetfulness is more likely to be a vascular lesion. Chronic headache may indicate the presence of a mass lesion while a sudden onset thunder-clap headache is suggestive of subarachnoid haemorrhage or meningitis. A sudden loss of consciousness suggests a brain haemorrhage, large infarct or a seizure while a more gradual deterioration is usually seen in metabolic, toxic or infectious aetiologies. *The recovery from loss of consciousness without any medical intervention is seizure until proven otherwise.*
One common pitfall in my practice is when the educated children give the history according to their understanding and at such ignore most of the salient symptoms. History in such cases should be taken from the live in relative or care giver. An eye witness is needed for collaboration in cases like seizures, forgetfulness and loss of consciousness a close relative. The temporal profile differentiates between an acute, sub acute and a chronic lesion.

Acute Lesions (less than 2 weeks)
In most cases of acute neurologic lesions, the symptoms are usually of less than two weeks in duration. In certain conditions, the symptoms may be more rapid. Common causes of such rapid neurologic symptoms which occur within seconds or minutes include seizure, channelopathy or a vascular event.. Seizures are the most dramatic in nature.

Sub acute Lesions (2weeks to 6 weeks)
These lesions also have a short temporal profile but are not as dramatic as acute lesions. They usually build up from days to weeks. They evolution may be smooth, step wise or crescendo. These sub acute lesions usually suggest an expanding or worsening lesion. Common causes of subacute lesions are infectious abscesses, subdural haematoma and tumors.

Chronic Lesions (months to years)
Chronic lesions are characterized by slowly progressive deteriorating symptoms without remissions. Common causes are ly

neurodegenerative disorders, chronic infections, gradual intoxications, and neoplasia. Progressive and symmetric symptoms often have a metabolic(chronic renal failure, hepatic failure and endocrine disorders) or degenerative origin.

Recurrent lesions
In some cases, there are recurrent episodic attacks of symptoms accompanied by rapid and complete recovery. This indicates repeated episodes of a single process as occurs with transient ischemic attacks (TIA), seizures, migraine, and multiple sclerosis. In the case of seizures and migraine the symptoms are highly stereotypical. TIAs may be stereotypical or have variable presentations. In multiple sclerosis, symptoms are not only recurrent but they also vary depending on the site of the lesion. In addition, the process may evolve to a secondarily progressive one. In such cases, there is only partial recovery from each attack.

14.22 Evolution and course of the disease
It is pertinent to define the evolution and or progression of the symptoms in order to determine the involved pathological process. Seizures for example are classically paroxysmal (sudden onset and sudden offset) and will abate. There are usually associated periods of lucid intervals in seizure disorders. Sudden onset severe headache followed by reduction or loss of consciousness usually signifies acute brain haemorrhage like subarachnoid haemorrhage (SAH) or intracerebral haemorrhage (ICH). Similar severe headaches however with associated neck stiffness but preceded by fever indicates an acute meningitis. Symptoms that worsen after exposure to heat or exercise may indicate conduction block in demyelinated axons, as occurs in multiple sclerosis (MS). A gradual evolution of symptoms over hours or days suggests a toxic, metabolic, infectious, or inflammatory process. Relapsing and remitting symptoms involving different levels of the nervous system suggest MS or other inflammatory processes while a chronic worsening of symptoms will suggest a chronic neurodegenerative disorder or a neoplastic lesion.

14.23 Types of Symptoms

Symptoms may be negative or positive. Again, this is important in determining the patho-physiologic process and subsequently the aetiology.

Negative symptoms
These are symptoms where there is reduction (weakness, numbness) or complete loss (paralysis, analgesia) of function. They usually imply a partial or complete failure of impulse conduction in the system. They are considered "destructive". Some examples are the weakness of the muscle in mononeuropathies, the sudden weakness or inability to speak in cerebrovascular disease. Recovery in these lesions is usually difficult.

Positive symptoms
Positive symptoms result from an exaggeration of a physiological phenomenon. Some positive symptoms are tingling painful, sensations, seizures or abnormal involuntary motor movements. They usually imply abnormal excessive discharges in grey matter or an imbalance in opposing pathways or systems. They are considered "irritative." These positive symptoms can be brief and very intense paroxysmal as in epileptic seizures or episodic as in trigeminal neuralgia or migraine. They can also be continuous: chorea, dystonia, nystagmus and tremor.

Secondary symptoms
Secondary symptoms are those symptoms referable to "mass effect." They occur as a result of the development of oedema or pressure on adjacent structures leading to new symptoms or an increase in the severity of the symptoms. Some examples are seen in worsening of the hemiparesis or reduction in consciousness in infarcts. This can also be caused by pressure or compression from the growth and or expansion of tumours. Worsening consciousness, and mid brain signs like respiratory abnormalities are seen in tentorial herniation when there is a mass lesion in the brain. Raised intracranial pressure and blockage of C.S.F. pathways also cause altered or worsening consciousness and blurred vision with papilloedema. The stretching of vessels and

meninges cause the headache and stiff neck seen in meningitis and subarachnoid headache.

14.24 Associated Features

The associated features are important in defining the aetiology. The association of fever usually indicates an infectious or inflammatory process. It could also be due to a malignancy, endocrine process or a connective tissue disorder. Hence in a person with severe headache and altered consciousness, a preceding history of fever will suggest cerebrospinal meningitis whereas an absence of preceding headache is more likely to be from brain haemorrhage(fever may develop later).

However, headache with a similar but slower temporal march of symptoms accompanied by, nausea, vomiting, or visual disturbance suggests migraine.

The association of slurred speech with weakness of one side of the body in the early hours of the morning is in keeping with an infarct. However, the association of slurred speech with ptosis and weakness of the proximal muscles occurring gradually will suggest a neuromuscular junction disorder. A history of a prior innocuous fall about six weeks earlier in an elderly man with gradual weakness of one side, difficulty in speaking and deterioration in consciousness is suggestive of subdural haematoma. In the absence of the history of fall, other aetiologies should be considered. Weight loss is usually seen in chronic disorders like chronic infections, connective tissue disorders and malignancies.

14.25 Further history

Past Medical History

Further history is also pertinent in the aetiology. The past medical history may indicate or signify a progression or complication of the prior diagnosis. A past medical history of hypertension is important in a person with a sudden blurring of vision or weakness of one side of the body. A previous diagnosis of cancer in a person with headaches and seizures may suggest metastasis to the brain. The prior diagnosis of Diabetes mellitus in a person with parasthesias and erectile dysfunction suggests Diabetic neuropathy. Changes in the personality and a decline in the cognitive functions in a person with a previous diagnosis of HIV will suggest HIV Associated Dementia.

Family and Social History
The family history should be properly explored. A family history of tremors in a person with bilateral tremors will suggest a diagnosis of benign essential tremors. The history of significant alcohol intake in a person with confusion and confabulation will suggest Wernicke Korsakoff's psychosis. A history of recent travel to an endemic area in a person with fever may be suggestive of cerebrospinal meningitis.

Important Notes

1. History remains the most important tool in localization of lesions

2. All symptoms arise from a focal lesion at one location. Always attempt to explain all the features from one pathological process. Double or triple pathologies may co-exist in rare cases e.g. Hypertension and Cancer.

3. If symptoms are bilateral and distributed over many body segments, consider a multifocal (e.g. multiple sclerosis), diffuse (E.g. metabolic, toxic, ALS) disorder or a systemic disease like infection or metabolic

4. In hemispheric lesions, the deficit is contralateral to the site of the lesion.

5. Most vertical tracts cross at one point or the other. The horizontal level of the lesion determines whether the deficit will be ipsilateral or contralateral.

References

1. Baliga R R: 250 short cases in clinical Medicine 3rd Ed Saunders 2001.
2. Ekeh Bertha C; Clinical Neurology made Easy 1st Ed USA 2018
3. Epstein RJ. Medicine for examinations 4th Ed Canada 2006
5. https://emedicine.medscape.com/article/1146199-clinical
6. Kasper DL, Fauci A S, Hauser S L, Longo D L, Jameson J L, Loscalzo J: Harrison's Principles of Internal Medicine; 19th Ed New York 2015
7. Lindsay K W. Bone I: Neurology and Neurosurgery Illustrated 4th Ed Edinburgh 2005
8. Ropper AH, Brown R H: Adams and Victor' Principles of Neurology 8th Ed New York 2005
9. Swash M, Glynn M: Hutchinson Clinical Methods 22nd Ed Edinburgh 2007
10. Walker HK, Hall WD, Hurst JW; Clinical Methods, The History, Physical, and Laboratory Examinations 3rd Ed Boston 1990
11. Zazulia A R. Neurological Diagnosis & Localization; https://neuro.wustl.edu/education/medical-student-education/neurology-clerkship/localization/

PART 3

BASIC INVESTIGATIONS OF THE NERVOUS SYSTEM

CHAPTER 15

LABORATORY INVESTIGATIONS

15.10 Analysis of the Cerebrospinal fluid

The cerebrospinal fluid (C.S.F.) is formed in the choroid plexus. The choroid is located within in the third, fourth and lateral ventricles. The C.S.F. circulates through all the ventricules in the brain and drains into the subarachnoid space. Thereafter, it is reabsorbed into the venous system of the dura matter. The C.S.F. serves several purposes. The first is protection. It also helps in the regulation of the intracranial pressure which is consequent on changes in cerebral blood flow. The total capacity of the C.S.F. in the adult is about 150 ml. Normal C.S.F. pressure is about 100 mm of water (with a range of 80–180mm/H2O) in the lateral horizontal position. The biochemical composition and microscopic content of the C.S.F. change with different diseases, conditions, or medications. Cerebrospinal fluid analysis is important in the diagnosis of may diseases of the central nervous system. It is the most important laboratory test specific for neurological disorders. The C.S.F. is collected from a procedure called lumbar puncture or spinal tap.

15.11 Lumbar Puncture

The first step in performing a lumbar puncture (LP) is to exclude raised intracranial pressure. Clinical symptoms of raised intracranial pressure includes history of headaches worsened by increased intra abdominal pressure, projectile vomiting and altered consciousness.

Examination findings include decerebrate posturing, relative bradycardia (increased blood pressure without a concomitant rise in pulse rate) and 6th nerve palsy. Other features are dilated pupils and papilloedema on examination of the optic fundus. Ideally, a cranial CT scan should be carried out to rule out raised intracranial pressure in all patients before a lumbar puncture. However, this is not always feasible in poor resource centers therefore doctors in such centers may have to rely on the clinical features noted above. Lumbar puncture is almost always contraindicated in the presence of raised intracranial pressure because of the risk of consequent transtentorial or tonsillar herniation. *This risk of herniation however is considerable when the papilloedema is due to an intracranial mass. It is much lower in patients with subarachnoid haemorrhage, pseudo tumour cerebri and cryptoccocal meningitis.* In these conditions, repeated lumbar punctures have been employed as a therapeutic measure. In patients with purulent meningitis, there is a small risk of herniation. This risk of herniation is therefore outweighed by the need for definitive diagnosis and commencement of proper management. Barring this last exception, LP should be preceded by a CT scan or MRI whenever raised intracranial pressure is suspected.

In cases where an LP is considered absolutely, LP is performed with the following precautions:

a. Use a fine bore needle (22 or 24)
b. If the pressure is > 400mm H_2O, Mannitol or urea should be administered after obtaining the sample.
c. Dexamethasone may also be given at an initial dose of 10mg then 4mg 6hrly. This will produce a sustained reduction in intracranial pressure.

15.12 Indications/Applications
Indications for lumbar puncture are as follows
1. Collection of cerebrospinal fluid for analysis
2. C.S.F. Drainage and pressure reduction
3. Administration of spinal anaesthesia, antibiotics and cytotoxic mediations
4. Injection of radiopaque substances

15.13 The Lumbar Puncture Procedure
Lumbar puncture is carried out under strictly sterile conditions. This will include hand washing and sterile linen. The doctor should don a mask and use sterile gloves. The site of the puncture must be well clear of the termination of the cord hence it is usually performed between the 3rd and 4th vertebrae in an adult. A line joining the iliac crests passes through the 4th lumbar vertebra. Therefore the inter-vertebral space immediately above or below this landmark can be used with safety. Lower spaces are used in

young children in whom the spinal cord may extend to L3/L4 interspace. Correct positioning of the patient is essential. The patient should lie on his left side on the edge of the bed with the spine fully flexed. The patient can also sit on the bed with a fully flexed back. The degree of flexion (knees to chin) is very important because it ensures that the vertebral interspinous spaces are opened to their maximum extent. *The patient must not slump.*

Clean the site of the puncture as expected in sterile procedures. Open the sterile packs, sterile bottles including a sterile bottle for glucose. Check the manometer fittings if available. Infiltrate the site of puncture with Lignocaine.

Insert the needle with the bevel facing upwards (parallel with the dural fibres). In the seated person, the bevel should face right side up. Thereafter, pass the needle inwards and somewhat cranially (or aiming towards the umbilicus). This will transverse through the supraspinous and interspinous ligaments and penetrate the dura which causes a distinct 'give'. Occasionally root pain is experienced if a root of the cauda equina is impinged upon, but usually these roots float clear of the needle. After this, withdraw the stilette and wait for the C.S.F. which is collected in three sterile bottles. Remove the needle after the collection and apply the dressing. If bone is encountered, withdraw the needle, ensure the correct position and reinsert the needle. A dry tap is usually due to wrongly placed needle.

The C.S.F. pressure can be estimated (normal, when lying on the side, 80–180mm C.S.F.). A block in the spinal canal above the point of puncture can be revealed by a test called the Quenckenstedt's test

Apply pressure to the neck in order to compress the internal jugular veins. At first, the veins are compressed one after another then both of them are compressed together.

This compression of the jugular veins reduces venous outflow from the cranium and raises the intracranial pressure. This results in the displacement of the C.S.F. into the spinal sac with a consequent brisk rise of the C.S.F. pressure by 100-200 mm/ H_2O which quickly returns to the normal pressure within seconds after the cessation of the compression. If there is no sudden rise, it may be because the needle is not properly placed. In spinal block, there will be a rise on compressing the abdomen but there will be no rise when the jugular is compressed. Recently however, the test is not used because of the advent of imaging techniques. Jugular compression should not be performed when an intracranial tumour or other mass lesion is present or suspected.

15.15 Other methods of C.S.F. collection

Cisternal puncture and Lateral cervical subarachnoid puncture
Cisternal puncture and lateral cervical subarachnoid puncture are also methods to collect the C.S.F. These however are too hazardous are rarely recommended. They may however be safe in the hands of an expert. LP remains the preferred procedure. The obvious indication is when there is a spinal block occluding the flow of C.S.F.

Ventricular puncture
Again this is rarely carried out.

V-P Shunt
The C.S.F. can also be collected from a tube that is already in the ventricles like the shunt, drain or pain pipe.

15.16 Complications of Lumbar Puncture
Headcahe is noted in about a third of persons after lumbar puncture. Pain or discomfort at the needle entry site is also common. Rarer complications may include bruising, meningitis or ongoing post lumbar-puncture leakage of C.S.F.

15.17 contraindications to lumbar puncture
The contraindications to lumbar puncture include posterior fossa mass, infected skin over the needle entry, coagulopathy and brain abscess.

15.20 Components of the normal C.S.F

There are many biochemical parameters and microbial organisms examined in the normal C.S.F. Normal C.S.F. has an opening pressure of 8-18cm /H_2O (80-180mm/ H_2O). It has a glucose level of between half and two thirds of the patient's blood glucose. For this reason, during a lumbar puncture for C.S.F. analysis, a blood sample is also taken to measure the plasma glucose concurrently. The C.S.F. Protein is 15-45mg/dL (0.15-0.45g/L) while Myelin basic protein is less than 4ng/ml. The Chloride level is 110-125mEq/L (110-125mmols/L). Glutamine is 6-15mg/ dL (410.5 - 1.026 micromol/L). Lactate dehydrogenase is less than 2.0 to 7.2 U/mL (0.3 - 0.12 microkat/L). There are no RBCs and the WBCs are less than 5of which all are mononuclear. There are no bacteria, antibodies, DNA of common viruses and cancerous cells.

15.21 Interpretation
The interpretation of the C.S.F. analysis is carried out in a step wise manner. Interpretation starts from reading the pressure from the attached manometer. Thereafter, the gross appearance is observed. Further interpretation is done after the analysis in the laboratory.

15.22 Pressure
The C.S.F. pressure is measured by means of a manometer. The first step is to place the patient in the lateral decubitous position as already described. This position aligns the patient's head with the puncture site. Thereafter, connect the manometer via a 3-WAY tap to run up the column and read the height. The normal value is 80-150mm/H_2O. In a scenario where the spinal needle has no attached manometer, a surge as the C.S.F. is collected suggests that the C.S.F. is under pressure.

Causes of increased C.S.F. pressure are as follows; Brain haemorrhage, tumors, stroke, aneurysm and high blood pressure and cerebrospinal meningitis.

15.23 Gross Appearance
The gross appearance of the C.S.F. is best examined by holding up the bottle against a white sheet of paper. Normal C.S.F. is crystal clear and colourless like water. Colour changes may be seen in some cases.

Colour

The C.S.F. may be hazy, turbid, milky or cloudy in bacterial infections, tuberculosis or metastatic lesions. The turbid nature is attributable to both the presence of bacteria and leucocytes. Opalescent C.S.F. is seen in Cryptococcal meningitis. Blood imparts a hazy colour but more red blood cells will give a pink to red colour. A traumatic tap may confuse the diagnosis. In order to distinguish between a traumatic tap and sub arachnoid haemorrhage, three serial samples are collected in different sample bottles at the time of the lumbar puncture. The differences are shown in Table 3 next page.

Table 3: Differences between SAH and Traumatic Sample

S/N	Feature	SAH	Traumatic Sample
1	C.S.F. Pressure	Increased	Normal
2	Colour	Uniformly stained in all three bottles	Gradually clear in subsequent bottles
3	Number of RBCs	Equal in all three bottles	Gradually reduce in the 2nd and 3rd bottles
4	Presence of clots	Not seen because the blood has been greatly diluted and defibrinated	Large volumes of blood will cause a clot or form fibrinous webs
5	Supernatant fluid	Xanthochromic after days because of haemolysis	Clear supernatant fluid if allowed to stand or after centrifuging N/B Very large bleeds (RBC>100,000/mm ^{3}) may be xanthochromic due to contamination with bilirubin and lipochromosomes
6	Number of WBCs	More WBCs(may be several hundreds) per 1000 RBCs due to the haemolysis and reduction of the RBCs	1or 2WBCs per 1000 RBCs

Xanthochromic C.S.F.

A yellowish tinge to the C.S.F. is called xanthochromia. It is caused by the degeneration of the blood cells in the C.S.F. which takes many hours to occur. Xanthochromia is seen after 12 hours and may persist for as long as two weeks. There are other causes of xanthochromic C.S.F. which includes severe jaundice like in kernicterus. Elevated C.S.F. protein from any cause also results in a faint opacity and xanthochromia. This requires levels of protein of more than 150mg/100ml. Other haemoglobin breakdown products like oxy haemoglobin also impart a yellow tint to the C.S.F. In addition, the C.S.F. may also be xanthochromic when there are blood clots in the subdural or epidural space. Meningeal melanosarcoma is another cause of xanthochromic C.S.F. because of the increased melanin.

15.24 C.S.F. Cellularity

The C.S.F. in an adult usually contains no cells. There may be about five (5) lymphocytes or other mononuclear cells/L.

An elevation of the WBC in the C.S.F. always signifies a reactive process to the bacteria or other infectious agents, blood, chemical substances, an immunologic inflammation, a neoplasm or vasculitis. It is important to differentiate neutrophillic and eosinophillic leucocytes with some techniques. This is because eosinophillic leucocytes are prominent in Hodgkin's disease, parasitic infection and cholesterol emboli while neutrophillic leucocytes are commonly seen in bacterial infections. Organisms like bacteria, fungi, echinococci and cysticerci can be easily identified on gram stain. Special staining technique like Zhiel – Nielsen stain used in the case of tuberculosis may be needed. An Indian ink preparation is used to differentiate between lymphocytes, Cryptococci and Candida. Some other special techniques can be used to identify tumour cell markers.

15.25 C.S.F. CHEMISTRY
Proteins

The protein level in the C.S.F. correlates well with the concentration of total proteins and different fractions in the serum though much lower levels. The C.S.F. protein however, varies with age and the level of tapping (lumbar, cisternal or ventricular).

Normal C.S.F. protein taken from the lumbar puncture is 15 - 45mg/dl (0.15-0.45g/L). The predominant fraction in C.S.F. is albumin like in serum.

C.S.F. protein elevation may be seen in the following conditions:
1. Bacterial meningitis: The C.S.F. protein reaches 0.5g/l or more. Viral infections have a lesser elevation in the range of 0.5-0.2g/L. The C.S.F. protein is markedly elevated in tuberculous meningitis to levels higher than 1g/L.
2. Guillain – Barre syndrome
3. Chronic inflammatory demyelinating polyneuropathy
4. Paraventricular tumours
5. Froin syndrome; caused by the blockade of C.S.F.

However, the C.S.F protein may be falsely elevated in traumatic tap, increased RBC and haemoglobin. In such cases it is pertinent to apply corrections as follows: In xantochromic C.S.F., for every 10^3 RBC counted subtract 1.1 mg/dL from the measured total protein concentration of C.S.F.

Causes of Low C.S.F. protein include the following conditions:
C.S.F. leakage
Meningismus
Meningeal hydrops
Hyperthyroidism
It can also be noted after a recent LP

C.S.F. protein fractions and C.S.F. IgG
In certain conditions, such as in multiple sclerosis, evaluation of total proteins in C.S.F. is not sufficient. There is a need to further evaluate the different protein fractions and various immunoglobulins. IgG immunoglobulins is produced by the plasma cells on both sides of the blood-brain barrier (BBB): within CNS and in the serum. Therefore an elevation of the IgG fraction of C.S.F. suggests damage of the BBB.

Albumin

Albumin is synthesized in the liver and reaches the C.S.F. via diffusion. Normal albumin concentration in C.S.F. is about 500 times lower than that of serum. Elevated level of albumin in C.S.F. is also associated with disruption in the BBB caused by trauma or inflammation. The integrity of the BBB is evaluated with the Quotient of Albumin (Q_{alb}) is calculated as follows:

$Q_{alb} = (Alb_{C.S.F.}/Alb_{Serum}) \times 1000$.

Normally, the Q_{alb} is less than 9 which reflects intact BBB: an increase reflects damage to the BBB.

The IgG index on the other hand, reflects damaged BBB. IgG index is calculated taking into account the concentration of albumin (Q_{alb}) and IgG in serum as follows:

IgG index = ($IgG_{C.S.F.}/IgG_{Serum}$) / Q-Alb

A rise in IgG index that is greater than 0.7 reflects active production of IgG within the C.S.F: the BBB is intact. A decreased IgG index reflects damaged BBB. Lesions that damage the BBB include stroke, tumors, meningitis and infectious abscesses.

Oligoclonal bands

The C.S.F. oligoclonal bands are a population of gamma-migrating globulins. Detection of oligoclonal bands is associated with multiple neurological conditions though especially important for multiple sclerosis

C.S.F. Transferrin

In normal circumstances, the type of Transferrin present in serum is only the sialated isoform (Beta -1).The C.S.F. nevertheless, contains the specific, desialated isoform, also known as tau protein/ tau transferrin or Beta-2 Transferrin. *This C.S.F.-specific band/isoform should not be detected in serum*; the detection in drainage fluids suggests that the specimen is contaminated with C.S.F. It is therefore an endogenous marker of C.S.F. leakage after head trauma with consequent rhinorrhoea or otorrhoea. Other causes are tumour, congenital malformation or surgery.

Glucose (Glycorrhachia)

The normal C.S.F. glucose concentration is in the range of 45-80md/dl. This is between half and two-thirds of the plasma glucose when simultaneously sampled. In general C.S.F. glucose levels below 35mg/dl are abnormal. Decrease in glucose levels is due to glycolysis and impaired C.S.F. glucose transport through the BBB. C.S.F. glucose is useful in differentiating between the causes of meningitis since there is reduced glucose in more than 50% of patients with bacterial meningitis whereas the level is normal in viral meningitis.

Causes of low C.S.F. glucose (hypoglycorrhachia) include the following:
Pyogenic meningitis
Tuberculous meningitis
Fungal meningitis
Subarachnoid Haemorrhage
Widespread neoplastic infiltration of the meninges
Sarcoidosis

C.S.F. Lactate

The lactate found in cerebrospinal fluid (C.S.F.) is predominantly produced by central nervous system (CNS) glycolysis and is at such independent of serum lactate. Causes of increased C.S.F. lactate concentrations include bacterial meningitis where there is a rise of >35 mg/dL while a value of 25-35 mg/dL is seen in patients with tuberculous and fungal meningitis. Others are cerebrovascular disorders, hypotension, hydrocephalus, traumatic brain injury and inborn errors of metabolism. The RBCs contain high concentration of lactate and LDH. Therefore, xantochromic C.S.F. can give a false positive C.S.F. lactate and LDH results. Elevated C.S.F. LDH is seen in intracranial haemorrhage and bacterial meningitis.

Others
Glutamine
Glutamine is the major way of removing toxic metabolites of ammonia from the brain. It is formed as a result of the combination of ammonia with a-ketoglutarate. Evaluation of glutamine in C.S.F. is important in children with coma of unknown origin. The normal glutamine concentration in C.S.F. is 8-18 mg/dL. Causes of increased glutamine are the conditions in which ammonia accumulates, such as in liver disease, inherited urea cycle disorders, or Reye syndrome.

15.30 C.S.F. Microbiology

15.31 Microscopic examination
Normal C.S.F. has either no cells or very few cells present. If the C.S.F. sample is crystal clear as described above, a small drop of undiluted C.S.F. is examined under a microscope and the cells are counted manually. There is usually no need to count the differentials when the number of cells is very few (≤ 5) as expected. The differential count however is carried out when the cells are more than five (>5 cells).

15.32 C.S.F. total cell counts

Red blood cell (RBC) count

Normally there are no RBCs present in the C.S.F. Their presence therefore may indicate bleeding into the C.S.F. or may indicate a "traumatic tap". The differences are highlighted in Table 3 above.

White blood cell (WBC) count

White blood cells are normally less than 5cells/µL in the adult. A significant increase in white blood cells in the C.S.F. is seen with infection or inflammation of the CNS.

Conditions associated with a reactive C.S.F. lymphocytosis include the following:

Meningitis especially Tuberculous
Syphilitic meningoencephalitis
Parasitic CNS infection
Multiple sclerosis
Guillain-Barré syndrome
Meningeal sarcoidosis
Polyneuritis
Sub acute sclerosing panencephalopathy (SSPE)

Conditions associated with C.S.F. monocytosis include the following:
Chronic or treated bacterial meningitis
Syphilitic, viral, fungal, amebic meningitis
Intracranial haemorrhage
Cerebral infarct
CNS malignancy
Foreign body reaction

Conditions associated with increased C.S.F. polymorphonuclear neutrophils include the following:
Bacterial meningitis
Acute viral meningitis
Tuberculous and fungal meningitis
Amoebic encephalomyelitis
Brain abscess
Subdural empyema
CNS haemorrhage
Leukaemia
Cerebral infarct
Malignancies
Previous lumbar puncture
Intrathecal+ chemotherapy
Seizures

15.33 C.S.F. Microscopy Culture and Sensitivity
The C.S.F microscopy with culture is a very important part of the examination. In collecting the sample, 1ml is usually enough for routine cultures which should be collected before the commencement of antibiotic agents: C. S. F. bacterial culture

yields the aetiologic agent in 70-85% of cases. This reduces by 20% after commencement of antibiotics. In cases of mycobacterium however, 5 mL is the required volume. The C.S.F. sample is collected with a sterile bottle and *should not be refrigerated*. Common causative organisms of meningitis in adults are Streptococcus pneumonia, Neisseria meningitis and Haemophilus influenza. Common viral agents are the enteroviruses. C.S.F. must be cultured as soon as possible because N meningitides, S pneumonia and H. influenza are fastidious and fragile organisms. Ideally, the culture should be done within one hour of collection of the C.S.F.

Gram Stain
Gram stain differentiates between gram positive and gram negative organism in bacterial meningitis as follows: Strep pneumoniae is Gram positive diplococci. N. meningitidis is a Gram negative diplococci that appears as a coffee-bean shaped which may also occur intracellularly or extracellularly in PMN leukocytes. H. influenza is a small pleomorphic Gram negative bacillus. Some organisms require special stains like the Zhiel- Neelsen (acid-fast stain) test for Mycobacterium Tuberculosis and Indian ink stain for Cryptococcus neoformans(sensitivity is 50 % but highly diagnostic if positive). .

Culture and Sensitivity
Culture of the aetiologic organism is the gold standard in the diagnosis of meningitis. Specific culture media are used to culture for the identification of different organisms. N meningitides and S pneumoniae grow on blood agar while H influenza grows on chocolate agar. Cryptococcus can also be cultured but isolating T pallidum is extremely difficult and time consuming (diagnosis is by C.S.F. VDRL). The culture for M. Tuberculosis takes several weeks and delays diagnosis. Viruses can also be isolated from the C.S.F.

15.34 Immunology tests

Antigen tests
Antigen tests are carried out for bacteria, viruses, fungi and multiple organisms. The C.S.F. bacterial antigen assay can detect the antigens of H influenzae, S pneumoniae, N meningitidis, E coli, and group B streptococcus. This bacterial antigen test is specific (a positive result indicates a diagnosis of bacterial meningitis). It also has the added advantage of detecting bacterial antigens after the organism has been killed by antibiotics. However studies have not shown its superiority to the gram stain.

Currently, there is a rapid assay for qualitative detection of antigens. The BinaxNOW S. pneumoniae antigen card can detect the organism in the C.S.F. with a 99-100% sensitivity and specificity. Hence it aids in the diagnosis or ruling out the commonest cause of bacterial meningitis. Antigen test however should go hand in hand with cultures.

Cryptoccocal surface antigen is reliable in detecting cryptoccocal infection. A false positive reaction however may be seen with high titres of rheumatoid factor or antitreponemal antibodies. Neurosyphillis can be diagnosed with the C.S.F. using both the nontreponemal and the treponemal antigen tests. The treponemal tests are more specific

Polymerase chain reaction (PCR)

Polymerase chain reaction is a laboratory technique used to make multiple copies of a segment of DNA. It is very precise and can be used to amplify, or copy, a specific DNA target from a mixture of DNA molecules. The use of PCR has been particularly useful in the diagnosis of herpes virus meningitis and enteroviruses. It is more sensitive than culture in enteroviruses and 94-100% specific. Amplification of DNA by PCR is particularly useful in detection of the tuberculous bacilli in the C.S.F.

Serology
Serology tests are not limited to the blood but can also be used in other body fluids like C.S.F. Serologic test is based on the principle that most acute infections will elicit a predictable

immune response. They therefore depend on occurrence of a rise in antibody titres. Serologic test for Lyme disease is also diagnostic

TABLE 4: C.S.F. Examination in some conditions

S/N	Pathology	Colour	Pressure	Glucose	Protein g/L	Cells
1	Bacterial meningitis	Turbid Green if purulent	↑↑	↓↓	0.5-1 g/l	1,000-10,000 WBC/L
2	Viral meningitis	Clear	N or ↑	N	0.25-0.5 g/L	5-300 WBCs/L Rarely >1000
3	Fungal meningitis	Clear May be viscous	↑↑	↓		40-400 Mixed cells/L
4	TB Meningitis	Slightly opaque with cobweb formation	↑↑	↓	>1g/L	100-600 WBCs/L Markedly lymphocytes
5	SAH	Xanthochromic or bloody	↑↑	N		>5000 RBCs/L
6	Cerebral Haemorrhage	May be bloody	↑↑	N		>200RBCs/L Higher in assoc ventricular bleed
7	Multiple Sclerosis	Clear	N	N	N or 0.1 g/L Oligoclonal bands	0-10 WBCs /L
8	Guillain-Barre's Syndrome	Clear	N	N	0.50-1g/L	N or few WBCs/L mainly lymphocytes Higher in cases of HIV

15.40 C.S.F. cytology

In C.S.F. cytology, a cytocentrifuged sample is treated with a special stain and examined under a microscope for abnormal cells. This is often done when a CNS tumour or metastatic cancer is suspected. The presence of certain abnormal cells, such as tumour cells or immature blood cells, can indicate what type of cancer is involved.

15.50 Anaesthesia and chemotherapy

Some medications are also injected into the intrathecal space through a lumbar puncture where they spread through the C.S.F.. In this way, substances that cannot cross the blood brain barrier are delivered and spread through the central nervous system where they can be active. These are mainly medications used for anaesthesia and chemotherapy.

Baricity is the comparison of the density of a substance with that of the cerebrospinal fluid. It is important in general anaesthesia. It is used to determine the spread of a medication in the intrathecal space.

References

1. Baliga R R: 250 short cases in clinical Medicine 3rd Ed Saunders 2001.
2. Harold Ellis: Clinical Anatomy 11th Ed Oxford 2006
3. Kasper DL, Fauci A S, Hauser S L, Longo D L, Jameson J L, Loscalzo J: Harrison's Principles of Internal Medicine; 19th Ed New York 2015
4. https://emedicine.medscape.com/article/2093316-overview#
5. https://emedicine.medscape.com/article/232915-workup
6. https://microbeonline.com/key-points-for-the-laboratory-diagnosis-of-central-nervous-system-infections/
7. Ropper AH, Brown R H: Adams and Victor' Principles of Neurology 8th Ed New York 2005
8. Swash M, Glynn M: Hutchinson Clinical Methods 22nd Ed Edinburgh 2007
7. Walker HK, Hall WD, Hurst JW; Clinical Methods, The History, Physical, and Laboratory Examinations 3rd Ed Boston 1990

CHAPTER 16

RADIOLOGIC INVESTIGATIONS

16.10 Plain Radiographs (X-rays)

Plain X-Rays of the skull and spine were once considered essential steps in the evaluation of a neurological patient. They were therefore ordered routinely. However, this value is diminishing as more sophisticated modalities yielding more elaborate information now exist. That notwithstanding, radiographs are still used as a cheap of diagnosis of ailments like Spondylolisthesis. However there is still the risk of exposure to radiation.

16.11 Skull X-Rays

Views
The standard views are the lateral as well as occipito-frontal (posterior-anterior) views.
The commonest views in the emergency unit are the lateral and frontal views. Other views are; Towne's view, Reversed Town's view, Occipito-mental and Sub Mental views.

Indications
Skull X-Ray is needed in the diagnosis of the following conditions:
Trauma
Infections of the bones
Tumours of the skull bones
Metabolic bone disease
Battering seen in child abuse
Multiple Myeloma
Dysplasias
Leukaemias

16.13 Interpretation
In the interpretation of skull X-rays, the following should be noted.

Calcifications
Intracranial calcifications may be physiological like in the falx cerebri, choroid plexus of the lateral ventricles, lens, dentate nucleus, lateral commissures, and the pineal gland. Characteristically, the normal calcification of the choroid plexus is located in the central area. However, the lateral displacement calcifications seen in the pineal gland may be a feature of subdural haematoma or other space occupying lesions. Abnormal calcifications are also seen in tumours like craniopharyngioma, meningoma and others.

Evaluation of masses

Intracranial masses can be evaluated with the skull X-Ray. They may show as focal calcifications like the meningoma and craniopharyngioma mentioned above. Neoplastic masses may also be seen as focal bone erosion. Furthermore, the pituitary fossa can be evaluated with lateral skull and cone sella radiographs to characterize any pituitary mass lesion. There may be an expansion of the pituitary fossa or an erosion of clinoid processes.

Fractures and bone Configuration
The skull X-Ray is a very important investigation in head trauma as it may show fractures in the skull base which are best seen with the sub mental –vertical view of the skull. Configuration of the skull may be misaligned in congenital abnormalities and some cases of trauma. This is appreciated in cases of platybasia.

Others
Generalized bone erosions are seen in cases of multiple myeloma. The presence of fluid in the paranasal sinuses is a feature of infection or a leakage of a C.S.F. especially in cases of head trauma. Focal bone hyperostosis is a feature of meningoma. All these mentioned examples highlight the usefulness of skull

radiograph despite modern sectional imaging tools.

16.12 Spine X-Rays

The spine is examined with the A-P and lateral views. The spine X-Rays are usually carried out in segments viz: Cervical spine, thoracic spine, lumbo-sacral spine. In interpretation of X-Rays, it is important to look at all the views available in a systematic manner. Plain films of the spine are useful in assessing the spinal vertebrae. They are usually indicated in back pains, neck pains, trauma and infections.

Coverage

The first step is to observe the segment of the spine that is visible on both views. Thereafter, check the alignment by following the corners of the vertebral bodies from one level to the next. Furthermore, examine the vertebral bodies. Normally, the disc spaces gradually increase from superior to inferior. Finally, examine the edge of image to note other structures visible and the soft tissue.

16.13 Common abnormalities of the spine

Degenerative disorders: This is seen as loss of disc height, sclerosis and osteophyte formation. Destruction of the vertebral pedicle and or the vertebral body are features a metastatic lesion. Destruction of the disc and vertebral end plate of are features of chronic infections like tuberculosis.

Arthropathy: Erosion and fusion of inter vertebral joints and disc spaces usually signify arthropathies. In ankylosing spondylitis, sacroilitis is an early feature and is considered the hall mark of the disease.

Congenital abnormality: The spine X-Ray is a cheap cardinal investigation in identifying congenital abnormalities of the spine. Common spinal abnormalities are scoliosis (lateral bending of the spine) and kyphosis (forward bending of the spine). Others are hemi vertebra, spina bifida and cervical ribs.

Spondylosis
Spondylosis, or osteoarthritic spine disease, typically and primarily involves the cervical and lumbosacral spine. Spine X-Ray may show prominent degenerative spine disease like osteophytes or combined disk-osteophytes.

Spondylolisthesis
Spondylolisthesis is the anterior slippage of the vertebral body, pedicles, and superior articular facets, leaving the posterior elements behind. Plain x-rays with the neck or low back in flexion and extension will reveal the movement at the abnormal spinal segment.

Trauma: In cases of trauma, there may be fractures of the vertebral body, transverse process and or spinal process. Normal C-spine X-rays do not exclude significant injury. Clinical considerations are of particular importance when assessing appearances of C-spine X-ray.

Soft Tissue abnormalities
Examination of the soft tissue is pertinent in spine X-Rays. The soft tissues and the para vertebral line may contain masses or abscesses. These para spinal and or psoas abscesses are very important features of infectious disorders like TB and Staphylococcal infections.

16.14 Angiography

Angiography/Arteriography

Angiography (*angio* vessel and *graphy* write or record) is a medical imaging technique used to visualize the inside of the blood vessels. It is a relatively safe procedure and extremely valuable in the diagnosis of aneurysms, vascular malformations, narrowed or occluded arteries and veins. It is also used in arterial dissection and angiitis.

16.42 Uses in Neurology
Cerebral and vertebral angiography are used in the following conditions; diagnosis of vessel occlusion, stenosis or plaque

formation and aneurysms. Others are arterio-venous malformation (AVMs) and compression or displacement of vessels. In recent times however, the use for angiography has been limited by the advent of CT scan and MRI due to better visualization.. MRA also has the added advantage of avoidance of ionizing radiation and nephrotoxic contrast agents. However, new endovascular techniques for the ablation of aneurysms, AVMs and vascular tumours still incoporate the use of conventional angiography. *In fact, conventional x-ray angiography is the gold standard for evaluating the precise anatomy of the AVM.*

16.42 Procedure

In angiography, the patient lies down in the supine position. The access to the blood vessels is gained most commonly through the brachial or femoral artery for the arterial system and the jugular or femoral vein for the venous system. The standard technique is to inject the contrast into the artery. A local anaesthetic is injected before the catheter is inserted into the femoral artery. Thereafter, a "guide wire: is used to manoeuvre the catheter gently the vertebral or carotid artery. This makes the blood to be visible on the x-ray images. The imaging is done using an X-ray based technique such as fluoroscopy. The recorded film or image of the artery is called an *angiograph*, or more commonly an *angiogram* and venogram for the vein.

Digital Subtracting Angiography (DSA)

Digital subtracting angiography is a fluoroscopy technique used in interventional radiology. In order to keep the patient still, a some cases, a general anaesthetic may be required. It clearly visualizes blood vessels in a bony or dense soft tissue environment. The subtraction of the pre-contrast film from the angiogram eliminates the bone densities thereby improving vessel definition. In recent times, DSA is done less routinely because of the advent of computed tomography angiography (CTA), which can produce the same 3D images while being less invasive and stressful.

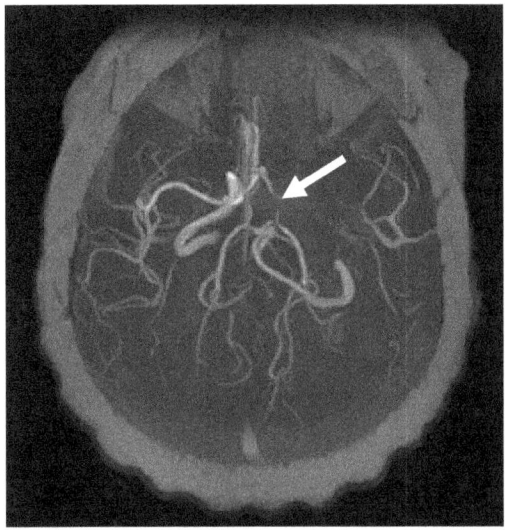

Fig 14: DSA showing occlusion of the left MCA

Uses in Neurology and Neurosurgery

Most neurological conditions require an accurate description of both intracranial and extracranial blood vessels. Another increasingly common angiographic procedure is neuro-vascular digital subtraction angiography which is used to visualize the arterial and venous supply to the brain. Intervention work such as coil-embolization and AVM gluing can also be performed.

Interventional Angiography

Interventional radiography is a rapidly developing field which provides new therapeutic options for patients with challenging neurovascular problems. It has led to a revolution in preventive neurology since intervention reduces the high risk of cerebral haemorrhage, stroke, or even death. Some of the available procedures include detachable coil therapy for aneurysms, particulate or liquid adhesive embolization of arteriovenous malformations and stent retrieval systems for embolectomy. Others are balloon angioplasty and stenting of arterial stenosis or vasospasm, and thrombolysis of acute arterial or venous thrombosis. There are still procedures for arterio-venous fistulae, venous malformations and tumours. The highest complication rates are found with the therapies designed to treat the highest risk diseases. There also some of these angiographic diagnostic and interventional techniques that is specific for the spine. Some of these are diskography, transforaminal and trans laminar epidural and nerve root injections, and blood patches.

16.20 Ultrasonography (USS)

The use of USS in neurology is mostly in the investigation of blood vessels, muscles and tendons. Ultrasonography can be used to form different types of images. The most well-known type is a B-mode image. This type displays the acoustic impedance of a two-dimensional cross-section of tissue. Other types of image can display blood flow, motion of tissue over time, the location of blood.

16.20 Advantages and Disadvantages

Advantages of USS
1. It provides images in real-time.
2. It is portable and can be brought to the bedside.
3. It is cheap and easily affordable.
4. It does not use ionizing radiation.
5. It is a safe non-invasive procedure.

Disadvantages
1. There is a need for patient cooperation
2. It has a high level of dependence on physique: the image quality is limited in obese patients.
3. The use of USS in the adult brain is very limited because of the difficulty in penetrating the skull bone.
4. Finally, the technique of USS is operator-dependent. Therefore results correlate with the skill and experience of the operator.

16.21 Uses in Neurology
Vascular USS
The most important use in Neurology is in angiology or vascular medicine. Duplex ultrasound is a combination of B Mode vessels imaging combined with Doppler flow measurement (see below). It is used daily to diagnose arterial and venous disease all over the body. The ultrasound is therefore used for assessing blood flow and stenosis in the carotid arteries (Carotid ultrasonography) and the big intracerebral arteries.

16.22 Procedure
The procedure of Ultrasonography in neurology could be used to examine both the extracranial or intracranial blood vessels.

Extracranial
The probe or transducer has a frequency of 5-10 Hz. it is applied to the skin surface. Ultrasonic waves emitted from various structures of varying impendence are detected by the probe. These waves are converted into electrical energy and displayed as a two-dimensional image (β-mode). Directing the probe at moving structures such as red blood cells within the vessel causes a shift of the waves. This shift is proportional to the speed of the flowing blood. This is called the Doppler Effect.

Doppler ultrasonography
Doppler ultrasonography is used to assess the movement of the structures like blood. It examines the movement towards or away from the probe, and its relative velocity. It employs the Doppler effect. Colour Coded Duplex (CCD) uses colour to super impose flow velocities on a two dimensional image. These are used to assess the external carotid and vertebral arteries.

Transcranial Doppler (TCD) and Transcranial colour Doppler (TCCD)
These techniques as earlier noted are used to measure the velocity of blood flow through the brain's blood vessels. In selecting lower frequencies (2MHz), ultrasound is able to penetrate the thinner parts of the skull. It is used in the assessment of intracranial

haemodynamics. It is also used to detect vasospasm in subarachnoid haemorrhage. Other uses are diagnosis of emboli and stenosis.

Musculoskeletal USS
Musculoskeletal ultrasound is important in the examination of muscles, tendons, ligaments, nerves, soft tissue masses, and bone surfaces. It is therefore useful in peripheral nerve and muscle disorders. In fact, quantitative ultrasound is an adjunct musculoskeletal test for myopathies in children.

16.30 Cranial Computerized Tomography (CT)

Computerized tomography is a non invasive procedure developed in the 1970's. The advent of this imaging technique revolutionized the investigative approach to intracranial pathology. Currently, it is routinely used for the skull and spine. Tomo means slice, cut or section while graphy means write or record. In essence, it entails the examination of the part of the body slice by slice.

The earlier name was computed axial tomography (CAT scan). This was because all the slices were axial initially. Most modern CT machines take continuous pictures in a helical (or spiral) manner. This is different from the earlier method of taking a series of pictures of individual slices of the body.

Helical CT therefore has several advantages. These include increased speed, better 3-D pictures. In addition, it may also detect small abnormalities better.

The newest CT scanners, called multislice CT or multidetector CT scanners, allow more slices to be imaged in a shorter period of time. In addition, these high definition views give sagittal and coronal reconstructions: hence axial was dropped from the name. It is therefore simply referred to as Computed Tomography (CT scan). However, the axial slices are still the more popular cuts and most CT scan pictures are axial. Computed Tomography is more than 100 times sensitive than the conventional radiography. However it uses ionizing radiation and at such requires same precautions as the conventional X-Rays.

16.31 Uses of Cranial CT scan

The cranial CT scan has numerous uses in Neurology. Topmost on the list is the diagnosis of cerebrovascular disease.

Diagnosis of Cerebrovascular disease (CVD)

The diagnosis of cerebrovascular disease remains the commonest and most popular use of the cranial CT scan. Ideally a cranial CT scan should be performed within 90 minutes after a CVD. The essence is to detect haemorrhage in the brain which is shown almost immediately by the cranial CT scan. Infarcts however will not be detected until after 48 to 72 hours. Therefore acute ischaemic stroke is ruled out by inference since acute CVDs are either haemorrhagic or infarcts. However, there are some subtle features which may be seen in early infarct. These are the loss of grey-white matter differentiation, asymmetry of the sulci and middle cerebral artery hyperdensity. Acute Haemorrhagic CVD like SAH, intracerebral or intraventricular haemorrhage will be seen as hyperdense lesions.

Detection of intracranial haemorrhage

Cranial CT scan is always very important in the diagnosis of intracranial haemorrhage (acute epidural and subdural haematoma) which all show as hyperdense lesions. It is also used in acute sub acute and chronic haemorrhage which will be isodense and hypodense respectively.

Detection of raised intracranial pressure

Cranial CT used to ascertain the presence of raised intracranial pressure before performing a lumbar puncture.

Detection of tumours and abscesses

Visualization of tumours, abscesses and aneurysms can be achieved with contrast enhanced CT scan. However MRI is more sensitive than CT scan.

Uses in Neurosurgery

The uses in Surgery include:

Evaluation of the volume of the ventricles after a V-P shunt
Evaluating facial and skull fractures in trauma
Evaluation of craniofacial and dentofacial deformities for surgical repair
Evaluation of tumours and cysts of the jaws and the paranasal sinuses
Evaluation of the nasal cavity as well as the orbits
Diagnosis of the causes of chronic sinusitis
Planning of dental implant reconstruction

16.32
Advantages and Disadvantages

Advantages

1. The CT scan is safe when metal is present in the body unlike the MRI which is a powerful magnetic field.
2. The CT scan gives clarity of blood from the moment of bleeding unlike the MRI.
3. CT scan is cheaper. It is also readily available and accessible especially in poor resource settings.
4. The examination time is shorter in CT scan.
5. The CT scan also has superior visualization of calcium, fat, and bone, especially the skull base and vertebrae.
6. The CT scan can be carried out during monitoring and use of life-support equipment.
7. Pts with Claustrophobia can undergo a CT scan but not an MRI.

Disadvantages
1. The CT scan utilizes ionizing radiation.
2. It does not visualize early infarction and lesions of the posterior fossa easily.
3. It has poor resolution for soft tissues and demyelination

The major limitation of CT is the presence of linear artifacts which result in "beam hardening" creating dense or lucent streaks that cross the brainstem obscuring underlying lesions.

16.33 Procedure
In performing a cranial CT scan, a pencil beam of X-ray is passed through the patient's head. Diametrically opposed detectors measure the extent of absorption. The absorption values are passed through computer processing and further reconstruction to produce the CT scan appearance. In CT, the effect of the X-radiation is reduced as it passes successively through the skull, C.S.F., cerebral grey and white matter and blood vessels. The intensity of the exiting radiation relative to the incident radiation is measured. For routine scanning, slices are 5-10mm wide. Recently slices can be as thin as 0.5- 1mm which provides better details.

Use of Contrast Medium
An intravenous iodinated water-soluble contrast medium is administered when the plain scan reveals an abnormality that requires more details. Occasionally, the contrast may be given orally or rectally. Contrast is also used when there is a specific indication like in suspected aneurysm. In spinal CT, a small amount of intrathecal contrast may be needed. The contrast is needed to highlight some features just as in other radiological investigations. Commonly used dyes are Iodine and Barium. The scans are usually labeled NCCT (Non contrast CT) or CECT (Contrast Enhanced CT).

16.34 Step wise interpretation

Interpretation of the cranial CT scan requires a step wise organized process just like most other investigations in Medicine. It is important to identify the scanogram in order to recognize the levels of the slices. Identify all the different views: axial sagittal and coronary views.

Orientation
The CT axial cuts are slice viewed as though the reader is looking up from the patient's feet. Thus, the left side of the scan is the viewers right and vice versa. The scanogram is at the top left corner. The upper part of the axial scan is the anterior part while

the lower part is the posterior part. It is important to ensure that the scan is square by noting that the orbits are parallel.

Terminology

The CT scan measures differing densities of structures. This density is seen in different shades ranging from white to black. The structures with a low density look *dark* while those with a high density look *white*. The terminology for CT scan is 'dense". *The more the density of the structure/lesion, the whiter it looks while the structures and lesions with low density are dark.* All structures and lesions are described as *hyperdense* (whitish), *hypodense* (dark), *isodense* (grey like the brain grey matter) and *mixed dense* (mixture of dark and white lesions. CT images are made up of pixels. Each of these pixels has a gray scale value. This value corresponds to the amount of X-rays that pass through the structure. It is also measured as well as expressed in Hounsfield units (HU). Using the HU to evaluate and quantify tissues, there are about 256 shades of gray that are indistinguishable to the naked eye. The HU values of different structures are shown in Table 5.

Table 5: Hounsfield units of different structures

S/N	Structure	Hounsfield Units	Colour
1	Cortical bone	+1000	White
2	Cancellous bone	+400	White
3	Blood	+50 to +100	White
4	Brain Parenchyma	+20 to +40	Grey
5	C.S.F.	0	Dark
6	Fat	-100	Dark
7	Air	-1000	Black

Contrast Enhancement
It is important to determine if contrast has been used. Lesions like haemorrhage do not need contrast enhancement. Infections and tumours however may not be obvious but will be highlighted to look white (hyperdense) when a contrast medium is injected. Contrast therefore can easily be mistaken for haemorrhage.

Principle of Contrast Enhancement
The BBB as earlier noted prevents substances from getting into the brain. The administered contrast therefore is unable to penetrate most of the structures in the brain. However, it will penetrate the blood vessels and structures lacking a BBB (e.g., the circumventriculo organs, pituitary gland, choroid plexus, and the dura) leading to a physiological enhancement of these structures. Pathologically therefore the iodinated contrast identifies both vascular structures and detects defects in the blood-brain barrier (BBB).

Pathologic lesions that cause contrast enhancement
1. All the lesions that break down the BBB
   a. Infectious processes(bacterial ,viral, fungal , protozoan and parasitic)
      Some examples include cerebral abscess, meningitis, toxoplasmosis, tuberculoma, cryptococcoma, chagoma, amoebic abscess, hydatid cyst, neurocystercercosis, and neurobrucellosis.
   b. Radiation injuries
   c. Contusion
2. Early infarct
3. Lesions with increased vascularity

All malignancies either primary or secondary will enhance because of the increased vascularity. Some examples include Astrocytoma, Glioblastoma multiforme, lymphomas, Kaposi sarcoma, Choriocarcinoma, Bronchogenic carcinoma, malignant melanoma and renal cell carcinoma.

4. Lesions in the vessel

Aneurysms, arteriovenous malformations, Cavengioma, Haemangioblastoma

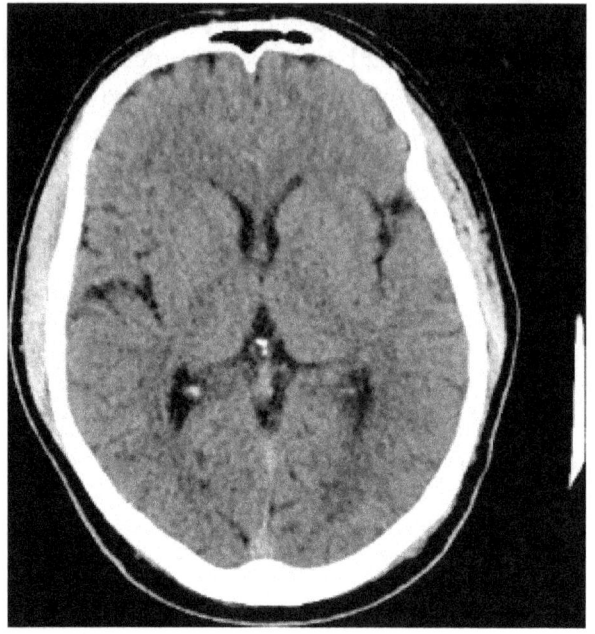

Fig 15 Normal Axial Brain NCCT scans

The pneumonic is for identification of pathological lesions in the cranial CT scan is "Blood can be very bad". The pneumonic represents the following:

B LOOD ; B for blood
C AN   : C for cisterns
B E   : B for brain parenchyma
V ERY   : V for ventricles
B AD   : B for bones

Blood

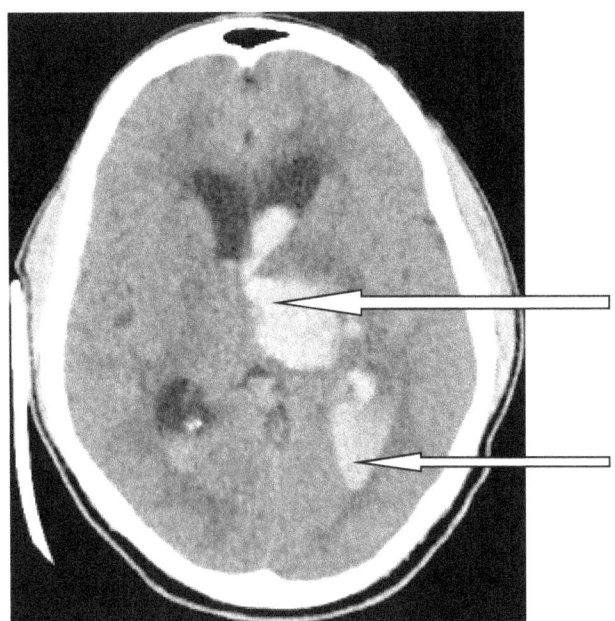

Fig 16 NCCT scan of left thalamic haemorrhage with intraventricular extension

Acute haemorrhage as shown in Fig 16 above appears hyperdense (white) on NCCT scans. This colour however changes with time. It becomes isodense over the following 1-4 weeks. Finally the bleed is hypodense over the subsequent 4-6 weeks. Hence acute haemorrhage is hyperdense, sub acute haemorrhage is isodense and chronic haemorrhage is hypodense.

The haemorrhage could be within the brain: intracerebral, intraventricular, and cerebellar or in the subarachnoid space as earlier mentioned. There could also be blood outside the brain but within the skull. This could be subdural haematoma which is usually concave or crescent- shaped and does not cross the suture lines but it crosses the midline. Extradural haematoma however is biconvex shaped and crosses the midline but does not cross suture lines.

Cisterns

Cisterns as noted earlier are collections of C.S.F., which surround and protect the brain. They contain C.S.F. and at such have the colour and Hounsfield value of C.S.F. It then follows that the normal cisterns should be dark in colour like the ventricles. In examining the cisterns, the first step is to note colour changes. The cisterns and sulci and fissures will appear hyperdense in subarachnoid haemorrhage in NCCT scans. Hyperdense cisterns, sulci and fissures however depict inflammation of the meninges in CECT scans. The aetiology may be infectious, chemical or neoplastic. In cerebral oedema or raised intracranial pressure there will be asymmetry or obliteration of the cisterns and sulci. Unilateral effacement is seen in pathologies involving one side while bilateral effacement is seen in bilateral lesions.

The circummesencephalic cistern which is located around the midbrain is the first to be effaced when there is raised intracranial pressure while the quadrigeminal is effaced early in rostrocaudal herniation. The star shaped suprasellar cistern is the most frequent site for aneurysmal SAH. Sylvian fissure is the site for traumatic SAH; it is also involved in mid cerebral aneurysms.

The cisterns and fissures may also be widened in hydrocephalous.

Brain parenchyma

The first step in examining the brain parenchyma is to look at the colour of the grey and white matter which are both grey in colour albeit different shades. The pathological lesions will be hyperdense, hypodense, isodense or mixed dense.

Hyperdense lesions

Hyperdense lesions as noted above appear white or whitish because they have a higher density than the brain parenchyma. These include blood, calcification, aneurysm, arterio venous malformations and harmatomas. The Hounsfield values of the different lesions as shown in (Table 3) will differentiate these different pathologies.

Hypodense lesion

Hypodense lesions are darker than the brain parenchyma. They may have the colour of C.S.F. All the lesions that have a density that is lower than that of the brain parenchyma will be hypodense.

Such lesions include infarction, oedema, tumour, encephalitis, abscess and resolving haematoma.

Isodense lesions
Isodense lesions are difficult to appreciate because they have the same grey colour as the brain parenchyma. Experience is required in isodense lesions. Often times, other features like mid line shift, obliteration of the sulci and fissures or enlarged ventricles aid in their recognition. Some examples of isodense pathologies include early infarct, oedema, sub acute haemorrhage and tumours.

Mixed dense lesions
Certain lesions have a combination of areas which are hyperdense and some others areas which are hypodense. Some examples of lesions with mixed density include abscess, arterio venous malformation, haemorrhagic infarct and contusion.

Symmetry
The sulci and gyri are usually well differentiated in adults. They are symmetric from side to side. On examination of the scan, it is pertinent to compare the sulci on the same position bilaterally. Sulcal asymmetry is seen in localized lesions, like infarcts and focal oedema. In generalized oedema (like after a generalized seizure) or viral encephalitis, there is generalized obliteration of the sulci.

Midline shift
In normal scans, the falx cerebri is located in the midline with the ventricles evenly spaced at the sides. A shift of the falx and ventricles to the side indicates the presence of a compressive lesion from the opposite side. This is seen in intracranial haematoma and mass lesions with oedema. Mid line shift is particularly important in isodense lesions where it leads the interpreter to look for the cause of the shift. Loss of cisternal space is an evidence of the rarer rostrocaudal shift.

Loss of Grey-White matter Differentiation
The outer grey and inner white matter which are best visualized in axial scans are both grey in colour. The shades of grey however

differ with the grey matter being a darker shade of grey. Occasionally the two areas seem to merge into each other and become the same shade. This is referred to as *loss of grey –white matter differentiation*. It is a classical feature of early infarct. It is also seen in metastatic lesions often found at grey-white border.

Ventricular system
The examination of the ventricular system yields valuable information and should be examined in the following order:
Size
The prominence of the ventricles is seen in hydrocephalus. Causes of hydrocephalous include intraventricular haemorrhage, migraine and obstructive hydrocephalous. Massive hydrocephalous with associated widening of the sulci and fissures depicts cerebral atrophy seen in dementia (Hydrocephalous ex vacou).
Position
The change in position of the ventricles and the presence of midline shift should be noted. The ventricles are moved to a side in mid line shift as noted above. An obliteration of the ventricle may be noted when there is obstructive hydrocephalous.

Colour
The ventricles contain C.S.F. and should be dark in colour with a Hounsfield unit of zero. The ventricles may be hyperdense when there is intraventricular haemorrhage.

Symmetry
There may be a normal variation in the sizes of normal ventricles. Such asymmetry occurs in as much as 5-20% of the population. Commonly, the right ventricle may be larger than the left. Significant asymmetry may suggest; compression of the ventricle, unilateral or obstructive hydrocephalous.

Bones
The last parameter to examine in the CT scan is the cranium. Bones are best visualized on CT scan. Some of the features seen are depressed skull fractures, bone erosions which may be focal (e.g. pituitary fossa tumours) or generalized (multiple myeloma).

Patients with meningoma and Paget's disease of the bone may have bone hyperostosis.

Bone Window
Windowing or gray-level mapping is the process whereby the CT image gray scale component of an image is manipulated via the CT numbers. This results in an appearance of the picture that highlights particular structures. Bone window images are routinely used to characterize different skull lesions being excellent for demonstration of skull tables and the diploic space. They are recommended in abnormal skull films, suspected congenital anomalies, presence of enhancing lesions in close proximity to skull bone and suspected metastatic disease.

Other issues
Multiple lesions
Certain lesions are usually multiple in presentations. Commonest causes of multiple lesions are abscesses, granulomas or cases of multiple infarcts. Others are tumours especially with lymphomas and secondary metastases. Toxoplasmosis characteristically presents as deep seated multiple lesions.

Calcification
The basal ganglia, pineal gland and choroid plexus may be seen to be calcified physiologically. Calcification is commonly seen in blood vessel disease like AVMs, harmatomas and arteriosclerosis. It also occurs in some infectious diseases like cystercercosis, hydatid cyst and cytomegalovirus (CMV). Neoplastic lesions also cause metastatic calcification.

16.40 Brain Magnetic Resonance Imaging

Magnetic Resonance Imaging is also an imaging modality in which the body is studied in slices. It was formerly called Nuclear magnetic resonance imaging which was changed to make the name more acceptable. It has the benefit of not using ionizing radiation. MRI provides better resolution of most structures making it the procedure of choice in most neurological disorders. CT provides good spatial resolution (the ability to distinguish two separate structures at an arbitrarily small distance from each other). MRI on the other hand provides comparable resolution. It has far better contrast resolution (the ability to distinguish the differences between two arbitrarily similar but not identical tissues).

16.41 Advantages and Disadvantages of MRI
Advantages
1. MRI selects any plane ab initio unlike CT that needs to have coronal and sagittal reconstructions
2. MRI does not use ionizing radiation like the CT Scan.
3. It gives better resolution of different structures. This makes it the investigation of choice for most neurologic conditions.
4. MRI shows the areas of demyelination (important in the diagnosis of inflammatory demyelinating diseases).
5. MRI also has the advantage of visualizing the spinal roots, spinal cord and cauda equina.
6. The MRI also visualizes the posterior fossa.
7. MRI has no bone artifacts.

Limitations of the MRI
1. MRI is expensive and requires a special MRI suite and cooling to contain the powerful magnetic field.
2. The scanning procedure takes a longer duration.
3. MRI has a decreased sensitivity in SAH.
4. The imaging of the bone is limited to visualization of the bone marrow only.
5. MRI is contraindicated in patients with claustrophobia especially the closed system
6. MRI is contraindicated in patients with metals (cardiac pace makers, and aneurysm clips defibrillators, prostheses and even, IUCDs) because of the danger of torque and dislodgement of metals from their original sites
7. MRI (the closed system) is not used in patients on life support.

16.41 Procedure

Magnetic resonance can be detected from several endogenous isotopes. Hydrogen is the most abundant element in tissues and also yields the strongest magnetic signal hence it is used in current technology. The MR image is therefore a map of the hydrogen content of the tissue which principally reflects the water concentration. In an MRI examination, the patient is placed in a powerful magnetic field with the z axis straight up, the x axis through the nose, and the y-axis through the left ear (the origin is in the center of the head). This will cause the isotope (hydrogen atoms) to align in the longitudinal orientation of the magnetic field. A brief application of radiofrequency (RF) pulse results in a shift of a small percentage of protons into higher energy states causing a change in the axis of alignment of the atoms from the longitudinal to the transverse plane. When the (RF) pulse which is applied repeatedly is turned off, the atoms return to their original alignment. The relaxation of these protons back to their original energy state is accompanied by the emission of radio wave signals. The absorbed energy results in a magnetic signal that is detected by electromagnetic receiver coils which is measured. Thereafter, the scanner stores the signals as a matrix of data which is subjected to computer analysis from which the image is constructed.

The rate of return to equilibrium of the perturbed protons is called the relaxation time. There are two relaxation rates. These rates influence the signal intensity of the image. They are referred to as T1 and T2 relaxation times. Modulation of the interval between RF pulses (TR) and the time between the RF pulse and the signal reception (TE) produces different images.

T1 Relaxation time (Spin –lattice)

The T1 relaxation time is measured in milliseconds. It is the time for 63% of the hydrogen protons to return to their normal equilibrium state. It depends on the time taken for the protons to realign themselves with the magnetic fields. Thus it is a measure of the rate of proton reorientation back to the Z-axis of the magnetic field. T1-weighted (T1W) images are produced by keeping the TR and TE relatively short.

T2 Relaxation time (Spin –spin relaxation)
The T2 relaxation also measured in milliseconds. It is the time for 63% of the protons to become dephased owing to interactions among nearby protons. It depends on the energized protons and their return to electromagnetic equilibrium. It is a measure of the interaction of protons during the relaxation process. The use of longer TR and TE times produces T2-weighted (T2W) images. The MR image thus is made up of a map of the distribution of hydrogen protons with signal intensity imparted by both density of hydrogen protons and differences in the relaxation time of hydrogen protons on different molecules. The differences in tissue T1 and T2 relaxation times enable MRI to distinguish between fat, muscles, bone marrow, and gray or white matter of the brain.

16.43 Interpretation
Similar to CT scan, a systematic approach is the best method for the interpretation of MRI. Once again knowledge of anatomy is of paramount importance. In interpreting the axial images it is wise to scroll through the MRI from bottom to top examining the different areas at a time.

Terminology

The terminology for MRI is *"intense"*. All structures and pathologies are described according to their signal intensity viz: high signal intensity (hyperintense), low signal intensity (hypointense), iso signal intensity (isointense) and mixed signal intensity (mixed intense).

T1 Weighted Images
T1 weighted images are useful for the brain parenchyma. Brain appears medium gray and CSF is dark gray, and air is nearly black(Fig 17). T1-weighted imaging is more sensitive to sub acute haemorrhage and fat-containing structures: *T1W highlights fat*. Therefore, fat and sub acute haemorrhage have high signal intensity on T1W images: white (hyperintense). Structures which contain more water, such as CSF and edema have low signal intensity on T1W images. This means that they lesion looks dark

(hypointense). Gadolinium contrast added to the T1 may "light up" a tumor or abscess. The enhancement is better with MRI.

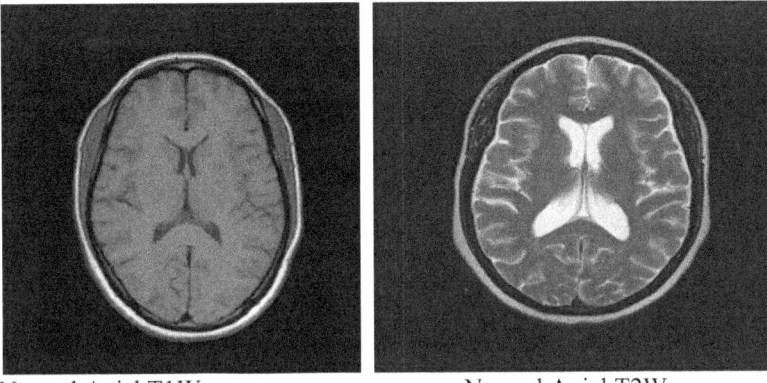

Normal Axial T1W   Normal Axial T2W

Fig 17 Normal axial Brain MR images

T2 weighted images

T2 weighted images are very good in the evaluation of the CSF spaces. The CSF appears bright white while the brain appears light gray. In essence T2W lights up liquids (Fig 17). T2W images therefore are more sensitive than T1W images to edema, demyelination, infarction, and chronic haemorrhage. All damaged tissues tend to develop edema; hence T2W is sensitive for pathology especially in multiple sclerosis, where it shows the characteristic periventricular white matter changes (bright splotches around the lateral ventricles). It is also very good in the evaluation of size and symmetry of the ventricles. Many other different MR pulse sequences exist. The selection of a proper protocol depends on the clinical evaluation.

FLAIR (Fluid –attenuated inversion recovery)

FLAIR is a sequence that produces T2W images in which the normally high signal intensity of CSF is suppressed (black in colour).It is therefore a (T2 with dark CSF).It highlights the areas next to C.S.F (periventricular areas) and areas near the cortex like multiple sclerosis (MS) plaques extremely well. FLAIR is also very sensitive to edema and parenchymal abnormalities like a low grade glioma. In fact a grade 1 astrocytoma will be virtually invisible on T1, but will be unmistakable on FLAIR. The main limitation is the poor quality in the posterior fossa and spinal cord.

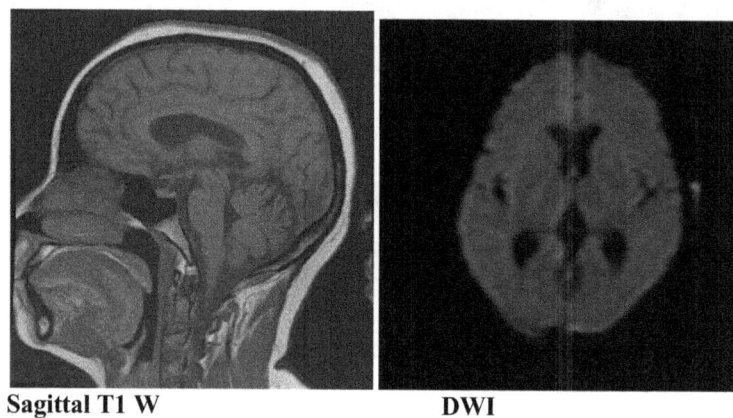

Sagittal T1 W   DWI

Fig 18 Normal Sagittal T1W and DWI MR Brain images

TABLE 6 Differences between T1W and T2W Images

S/N	S/N	T1	T2
1	Grey Matter	Grey	Black
2	White Matter	White	Black
3	C.S.F.	Black	White
4	Oedema	Black	White
5	Calcium	White	Dark
6	Fat	White	Grey
7	Air		Black
8	Acute Haemorrhage	Dark	Dark
9	Subacute Haemorrhage	White	White
10	Chronic Haemorrhage	Black	Dark
11	Subacute Thrombus	White	White
12	High Protein	White	Dark
13	Low Protein	Dark	
14	Gliosis		White
15	Metal		Dark

16.44 Paramagnetic Enhancement
The administration of gadolinium which is a paramagnetic agent enhances the process of proton relaxation. This is especially during the T1 sequence. This will cause a sharper definition and highlights many types of lesions. Most lesions that are markedly enhanced are lesions that break down the blood brain barrier in the brain, spinal cord or the nerve roots.

16.45 Other imaging techniques
Spin density–weighted imaging
The C.S.F. in this study has a density similar to brain tissue

Echo planar
Echo-planar is an extremely rapid MRI of the brain: in fact the fastest. It is capable of acquiring an entire MR image in only a fraction of a second (100ms/slice). The information for the entire brain is therefore obtained in 1 to 2 min, depending on the degree of resolution required or desired. However, the spatial resolution is limited.

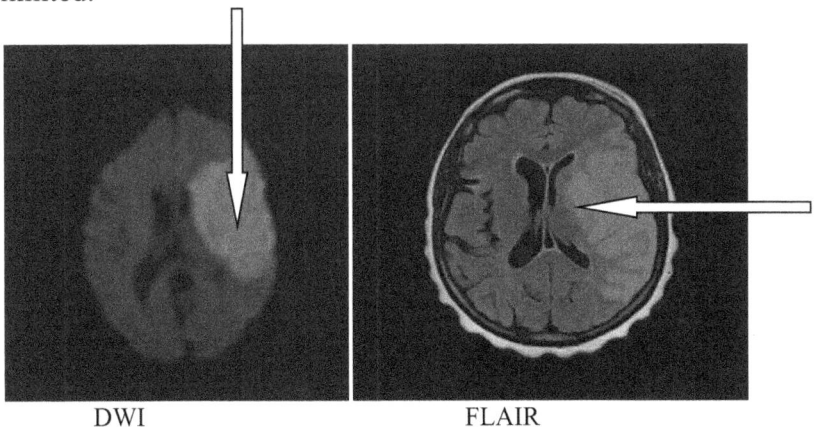

DWI   FLAIR

Fig 19 . DWI and FLAIR scans of ischaemic infarcts

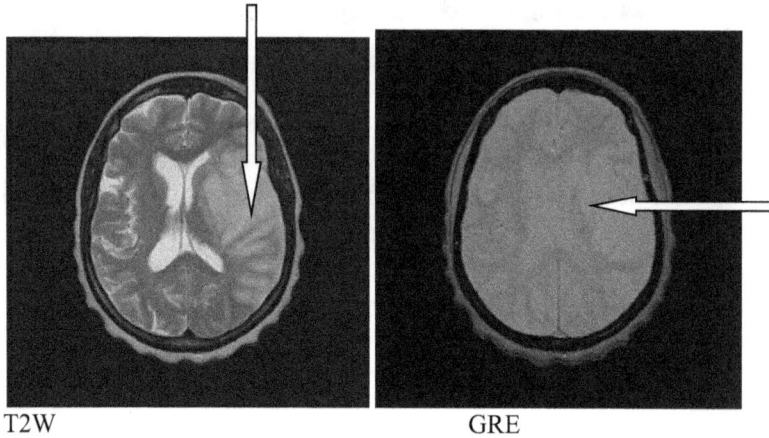

Fig 20 T2W and GRE MRI scans of ischaemic infarct

Diffusion-weighted imaging (DWI)

DWI uses the diffusion of water molecules hence; the images reflect microscopic random motion of water molecules. It calculates the apparent diffusion coefficient (ADC) which can be displayed on a separate screen. *It gives a high signal in acute ischaemic stroke within 10- 20 minutes and at such it is the initial imaging modality for acute ischaemic stroke when available(Fig 22).* It also gives high signal intensity in encephalitis and focal seizures. Other uses are the localization of cognitive functions.

Perfusion-weighted imaging (PWI)

Perfusion weighted imaging is a haemo dynamically weighted MR sequences are based on passage of MR contrast through brain tissue. It therefore gives information about the perfusion status of the brain. Bolus-contrast tracking is the technique that is used commonly most cases. It is based on the monitoring of a non diffusible contrast material (gadolinium) passing through brain tissue. The signal intensity declines as contrast material passes through the infarcted area and returns to normal as it exits this area.

The combination of DWI and PWI is superior to conventional MRI. This is so in both in early phases as well as 48 hours after the onset of stroke. This is because together they provide information about location and extent of infarction within minutes of onset. When performed in series, they also provide information about the pattern of evolution of the ischaemic lesion. This is of great importance in choosing the appropriate treatment modality, predicting outcome and prognosis.

16.46 Magnetic Resonance Angiography (MRA)

MR angiography is a non invasive procedure that highlights vascular anatomy and relationships. *The MR techniques used provide a vascular flow map rather than the anatomic map shown by conventional angiography.*

Uses of MRA

1. It is used in the evaluation of the extra cranial carotid and vertebral circulation
2. It is also used to assess larger-caliber intracranial arteries and dural sinuses
3. It is important in noninvasive detection of intracranial aneurysms and vascular malformations
4.

Limitations

1. It is lower in spatial resolution compared with conventional film-base angiography.
2. The detection of small-vessel detail as in vasculitis is problematic.
3. There may be motion artifacts.

There are two MRA techniques: Time-of-flight and Phase contrast.

Time-of-flight (TOF)

Currently, this is the technique most frequently used. It relies on the suppression of non moving tissue to provide a low-intensity background and does not require contrast. It shows the high signal intensity of flowing blood thereby highlighting arterial or venous structures. It is a flow based technique hence the main limitation is the over estimation of the length of occlusion or stenosis of the vessel. Tortuous or kinked vessels may therefore be considered stenosis.

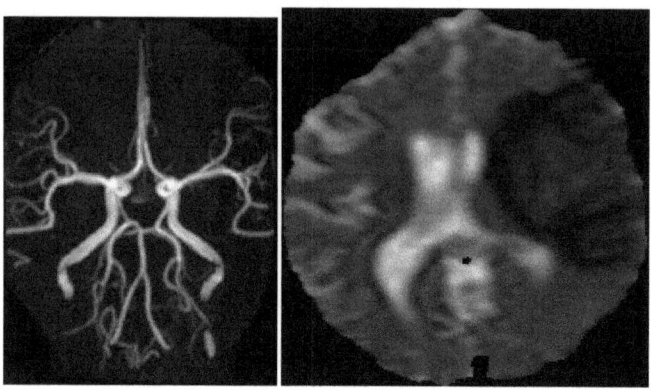

Normal 3D MRA   ADC
Fig 21. MRA Images

Phase- Contrast

Phase- contrast is an MRI technique that can be used to visualize moving fluid. It is typically used for MR venography. It does not require -IV-contrast. One limitation of TOF-MRA is in-plane flow voids. This does not limit the phase contrast. It is therefore helpful specifically in differentiating slow and absent flow from normal flow because *it captures only truly patent vessels.*It also reveals the velocity and direction of blood flow in a given vessel. One advantage is the excellent suppression of high signal intensity background structures. However, it requires a longer acquisition time than TOF MRA.

MR Spectroscopy

MR spectroscopy is a noninvasive procedure used in the assessment of chemical abnormalities in body tissues such as the brain. The main chemicals are choline and *N*-acetyl aspartate (NAA). Choline is contained mainly in cell membranes of myelin while NAA is a marker for neurons.

It also detects the breakdown products of Myelin. It can therefore distinguish a lesion due to infarct or tumor from demyelination. It is also important in diagnosis of HIV, CVD, head injury, coma, Alzheimer's disease, tumors, and multiple sclerosis.

Positron Emission Tomography (PET Scan)

This is a special technique that measures the regional cerebral concentrations of metabolic activity. It relies on the detection of positrons emitted during the decay of an injected nucleotide. The most frequently used nucleotide is 2-fluoro-2-deoxy-D-glucose(FDG). This is an analogue of glucose. It is taken by cells competitively with 2-deoxyglucose. There are multiple images of glucose formed after about an hour. The images therefore reveal differences in regional glucose activity among normal and pathologic brain structures. Alzheimers disease has been associated with a low activity of FDG in the parietal lobes. Reduced metabolism in the thalamus and the basal ganglia have also been noted in ADC. FDG PET is mostly used for the detection of extracranial metastatic disease.*Single Photon Emission Computed Tomography* assesses cerebral perfusion. It can differentiate between abcess and lymphoma.

16.50 Myelography
Myelography is a type of radiographic examination used in the investigation of the spinal cord. It uses a contrast medium to detect pathology of the spinal cord, including the location of a spinal cord injury, cysts, and tumors. It used to be carried out with X-Rays. In recent times however, the advent of MRI has made this investigation almost obsolete. This is because MRI has many advantages and does not require contrast fluid to be injected into the spine. CT myelogram is still carried out in persons who cannot have an MRI.

16.60 Interventional neuroradiology
Interventional neuroradiology is a rapidly developing field. It is particularly important in multiple cranial and spinal vascular pathologies. The procedures are minimally invasive and are used to diagnose and treat intracranial aneurysms and side effects of a subarachnoid hemorrhage. Other intracranial and spinal vascular disorders include Arteriovenous

Malformations, Dural Arteriovenous Fistulae, Arteriovenous Fistulae, Tumors, Carotid Stenosis and Stroke in a broad range of the population.

Endovascular Embolization and Stenting

Endovascular embolization is a procedure used to treat cerebral aneurysm, vascular malformations, and certain tumors. It acts as an alternative to open surgery (craniotomy) when dealing with aneurysms. However, the embolization of an arterio-vascular malformation (AVM) is a helpful adjunct for subsequent open surgery and/or radio surgery. The procedure entails placing a thin braided cylindrical mesh (Pipeline embolization device) in the blood vessel to occlude or block off blood flow in the vessel, thereby preventing bleeding and rupture.

References
1. Ekeh Bertha C; Clinical Neurology made Easy 1st Ed USA 2018
2. https://en.wikipedia.org/wiki/Angiography
3. Houston H, Rowland LP; Meritt's Neurology 10th Ed USA
4. Kasper DL, Fauci A S, Hauser S L, Longo D L, Jameson J L, Loscalzo J: Harrison's Principles of Internal Medicine; 19th Ed New York 2015
5. Lindsay K W. Bone I: Neurology and Neurosurgery Illustrated 4th Ed Edinburgh 2005
6. Nwafor N N: Unpublished collection of Radiographic Images
7. Ropper AH, Brown R H: Adams and Victor' Principles of Neurology 8th Ed New York 2005
8. Swash M, Glynn M: Hutchinson Clinical Methods 22nd Ed Edinburgh 2007

CHAPTER 17

ELECTRODIAGNOSTIC TESTS

17.10 Electroencephalography (EEG)

Electroencephalography is the recording of electrical activity along the scalp. It measures voltage fluctuations resulting from ionic current flow within the neurons of the brain. In clinical contexts, EEG refers to the recording of the brain's spontaneous electrical activity over a short period of time usually only 20-40 minutes. The EEG plays a central role in the diagnosis and management of seizures. It is relatively cheap and convenient.

17.11 Indications of EEG

Diagnosis and Management of Epilepsy
The most important use of EEG remains the diagnosis of epilepsy. The presence of abnormal, repetitive, rhythmic activity having an abrupt onset and termination and a characteristic evolution defines seizure activity and at such clearly establishes the diagnosis. However, the absence of these abnormal findings does not exclude a seizure disorder. Classic abnormal findings on EEG are commoner during a generalized tonic clonic seizure than during the inter ictal period. The video- EEG telemetry captures the ictal episodes and thereby increasing the yield of positive EEG diagnosis of seizures. Abnormal inter ictal discharges may also be present in the absence of a seizure disorder. Notably, certain abnormal wave forms in inter ictal EEG are particularly characteristic of a seizures disorder. Some examples include hypsarrhythmia and 3 spike and wave discharge which is pathognomonic for absence seizures.

EEG is also required to characterize the seizure type prior to the selection of antiepileptic medications. It distinguishes seizures from other paroxysmal neurological events such as psychogenic non-epileptic seizures, syncope (fainting) and migraine variants.

Other uses in epilepsy includes assessing the risk of recurrence after an unprovoked seizure, predicting the likelihood of seizure relapse if medication is withdrawn and identification of epileptogenic region in epilepsy surgery candidates. Furthermore, the EEG is necessary in the decision to wean off anti-epileptic medications.

Sleep disorders

Polysomnography is the continuous recording of some electrophysiologic parameters to define sleep and wakefulness. The parameters are electroencephalogram (EEG), the electrooculogram (EOG—a measure of eye-movement activity), and the surface electromyogram (EMG) measured on the chin, neck, and legs.

Coma

The EEG is important in persons with coma. It helps in the diagnosis of metabolic encephalopathy where the classical triphasic waves are seen. In severe metabolic coma, occasional slow waves (delta) waves may be seen in EEG. The EEG is also used in monitoring the convulsive state and the detection of non-convulsive state in status epilepticus. Finally the EEG is used in predicting the prognosis in coma.

Diagnosis of brain death

The EEG serves as an adjunct test in the confirmation of brain death. In brain death there is electro-cerebral silence.

Other uses

1. Investigation of cognitive decline
2. Differentiating "organic" encephalopathy or delirium from primary psychiatric syndromes such as catatonia
3. Diagnosis of tumour (was once first line)
4. Monitoring the depth of anaesthesia
5. Monitor Amobarbital effect in Wada test

17.12 Limitations

The EEG is laden with many concerns that make it unpopular. Some of these are as follows:

Poor coverage

The EEG recordings mostly reflect the summation of EPSPs and IPSPs in the pyramidal neurons in the more superficial layers of the cortex. Large areas of cortex have to be activated synchronously to generate enough potential. Significant amounts of cortex, especially in basal and mesial areas of the hemispheres, are not covered by standard electrode placement.

Sensitivity and Specificity

It is important to note that a normal EEG does not necessarily exclude epilepsy. This is because some of the patients with epilepsy never show epileptiform discharges.

Secondly, an abnormal EEG demonstrating inter epileptiform discharges (IED) does not in itself indicate that an individual has a seizure disorder. In fact, IEDs are seen in some (0.5%) normal subjects who never develop epilepsy. IED may also be seen in other neurological disorders. In fact sensitivity (true positives) for diagnosis in epilepsy ranges between 25–56% while specificity (true negatives) is clearly better, but still variable at 78–98%. *In essence, absence of epileptiform activity is specific, but presence of epileptic activity is not sensitive for diagnosis of epilepsy.* These wide ranges can be explained partly by diverse case selection.

Other limitations

The EEG is of no use in the diagnoses of psychiatric illnesses. In addition, it has a limited effectiveness in research. This is because it records only a small sample of electrical activity from the surface of the brain. Furthermore, many of the more complex functions of the brain cannot be related closely to EEG patterns.

17.13 Procedure

The EEG is recorded by placing many electrodes on surface of the brain or the scalp. It makes use of many electrodes. The electrodes are 8-32 pairs in most cases. Each pair of electrodes transmits a signal to one of several recording channels of the electroencephalograph. This signal is made up of the difference in the voltage between the pair. The rhythmic fluctuation of this potential difference is shown as peaks and troughs on a line graph by the recording channel. The electroencephalogram (EEG) is essentially a voltage-versus-time graph and is recorded as a number of parallel wavy lines. These wavy lines also called *channels* represent the electrical potential between two electrodes. The channels are arranged for viewing into standard *montages* which compare the activity from one region of the cerebral cortex to that from the corresponding region of the opposite side. The current digital recording provides many more channels than the earlier type as well as flexibility in viewing the result.

Patients are usually examined with their eyes closed and relaxed on a chair or bed. Hyperventilation, light and sleep are used to bring to light some specific discharges.

17.14 Interpretation

Interpretation of the EEG is very challenging because of the noted issues with sensitivity. However, there are certain factors are known to guide the interpretation.

1. Children are more likely to have IEDs than older subjects.
2. IED is commoner in some certain types of seizures or epilepsy syndromes.
3. Location of an epileptogenic zone (temporal and frontal) is more significant than in the occipital zone.
4. Abnormalities of background cerebral rhythms, focal slow activity or regional attenuation are not specific.
5. Some types of epileptiform phenomena e.g. 3 per second spike wave discharge, Hypsarrhythmia and generalized photo paroxysmal response are strongly correlated with clinical epilepsy.
6. Frequent (one /month) seizures are more likely to have IED than those with rare (one /year) attacks.
7. Timing of EEG recording may be important e.g. an investigation done within 24 hours of a seizure is more likely to have epileptiform discharges than one carried out weeks later.
8. Some patients show discharges mainly in sleep, or there may be circadian variation as in idiopathic generalized epilepsies

9. Co-medication may be relevant, particularly drugs that lower seizure threshold or may themselves induce epileptiform activity.

17.15 Normal EEG Wave forms

The normal background waveforms are classified according to their frequency, amplitude, shape and sites. The EEG wave forms are as follows:
Alpha waves ------- 8-13 Hz
Beta waves ---------- > 13 Hz
Theta waves---------- 3.5-7.5 Hz
Delta waves ---------- 3 Hz or less

Alpha waves are seen in a normal fully conscious adult who is relaxed. The waves are regular, recurring as well as oscillating. They are replaced by rapid irregular low-voltage waves in times of excitement or startle. During sleep, the brain waves become extremely slow. Slow waves are also seen in deep coma as well as other abnormal conditions.

Alpha (α) waves

Alpha waves have a frequency of 8-13 Hertz (cycles/second). It is seen in all age groups but is most common in the fully conscious adult as already noted and disappear with mental activity (arithmetic, stress, and thinking). In essence, they are prominent with the eyes closed and attenuate with attention and mental activity. Morphologically, they are rhythmic, regular, and waxing and waning. They are usually bilateral and are more obvious in the occipital and parietal areas. The amplitude of the wave however is higher on the non dominant side especially in right-handed individuals. The amplitude is generally 20-100 mV. Alpha waves are normal in most instances but are abnormal in alpha coma and hypoxic-ischaemic encephalopathy.

Beta (β) waves

Beta waves are the fastest of all the wave forms with a frequency of 13 to 30Hz. They are located mostly in the frontal and central areas of the cerebral cortex. Beta waves are also observed in all age groups but are obvious at the onset of sleep in infants more than 6 months. Morphologically, they are usually symmetric, rhythmic, waxing and waning. . The amplitude is small with a range of 5-20 mV. Sedatives like benzodiazepines and barbiturates augment the beta waves while voluntary movements and proprioceptive stimuli attenuate these waves. The amplitude can be mildly different (<35%) between the two hemispheres. A significant difference in amplitude (at least 50%) is abnormal. A higher difference may suggest skull defect while lower amplitude usually indicates a structural lesion.

Theta (θ) waves
These are slow waves with a frequency of more than 3.5 -7.5 Hz. It is normally seen in sleep (especially light sleep in an adult) at any age. Theta waves seen in a wake adult is abnormal. Theta and delta waves are referred to as slow waves.

Delta (δ) waves
Delta waves are the slowest of all the waves with a frequency of 3Hz or less. They have the largest amplitude also. They are normal in deep sleep in adults in infants and children. It is abnormal to see them in the wake adult. Delta waves can be seen in specific sites when there is focal pathology or diffuse in generalized dysfunction. Delta waves are commonly seen in the late stages of hepatic encephalopathy.

Others
Other less commonly recognized waves are sleep spindles, v waves, lambda waves, mu waves and the k complex.

17.16 Interictal Epileptiform discharges

The International Federation of Societies for Electroencephalography and Clinical Neurophysiology (IFSECN) describes interictal discharges as a subcategory of "epileptiform pattern". Epileptiform waves are "distinctive waves or complexes, distinguished from background activity, and resembling those recorded in a proportion of human subjects suffering from epileptic disorders. They are as follows:

Sharp waves
Sharp waves are transient and are clearly distinguishable from background activity. They have a pointed peak at conventional paper speeds and duration of 70-200 milliseconds (ms).

Spikes
Spikes are similar to sharp waves but have duration of between 20 and 70 ms (narrower) than the sharp waves.

Spike-and-slow-wave complex
The spike and slow wave pattern is made up of a spike followed by a slow wave (classically the slow wave being of higher amplitude than the spike). In some cases they may be multiple such that there are two or more spikes associated with one or more slow waves *(multiple spike and slow wave complex)*.

Triphasic waves
These are high-amplitude (>70 µV), positive sharp transients. They are preceded and followed by negative waves of relatively lower amplitude (three phases i.e. "low negative" then "high positive" and "another low negative"). They are diffuse and bilaterally synchronous with a typical bi frontal predominance. Another characteristic is they are usually repeated. The repetition is at a rate of 1-2 Hz. Triphasic waves are classically seen in metabolic encephalopathies.

Burst Suppression
Burst suppression is made up of bursts of activity (mixture of sharp and slow waves) which are periodically interrupted by suppression (activity of <10uV). Typically, the episodes of suppression (4-10seconds) are longer than periods of bursts (1-3) seconds. Burst suppression is typically caused by anoxic injuries, high doses of sedatives e.g. Barbiturates, Benzodiazepines and Protocol.

Alpha coma
The alpha wave has already been described as a wave that is prominent with relaxation, attenuates with attention and more obvious posteriorly. In alpha coma however, there is an

unremitting alpha activity that is unresponsive to eye opening, mental activity or other stimulation. It is monorhythmic, diffuse and uniformly distributed (equal amplitudes anteriorly and posteriorly). Alpha coma is seen in hypoxic-ischemic encephalopathy and destructive processes.

17.17 Characteristic Interictal Abnormalities
Much as the EEG may not be sensitive, certain abnormal waves are highly suggestive of epilepsy. These are characteristic or pathognomonic of certain conditions.

Hypsarrhythmia
There are disorderly high voltage waves which are asynchronous and chaotic. They are characteristically associated with West syndrome.

3 –per -second spike and wave complexes
The 3-per-second spike-and wave complexes are diagnostic of absence seizures. These are spike and wave complexes that occur three per second in a normal EEG background. They characteristically appear in all leads of the EEG simultaneously and disappear almost as abruptly as they appeared signifying the end of the seizure.

Electro cerebral Inactivity (ECI)
Electro cerebral inactivity is an activity that is not greater than 2 µv. The recording of ECI must be according to strict guidelines. The guidelines require a specific recording time. Another requirement is the doubling of the distances between the electrodes. They also ensure the reactivity of the testing, as well as the integrity of the system. ECI almost always results from profound cerebral hypoxia, ischaemia, trauma or raised intracranial pressure. In severe cases, there is no brain activity at all. This is called Electro cerebral silence is the most pathologic finding of all. It means that the electrical activity is absent. The EEG looks in like straight horizontal lines. It is a feature of brain death. Other features of brain death are absent brainstem reflexes, absent spontaneous respiratory. Loss of muscular activity of any kind for

6 hours is also a sign. The brain of such a patient is largely necrotic, and there is no chance of neurologic recovery.

17.20 Evoked Potentials

Evoked potential is the noninvasive recording of spinal or cerebral potentials which is elicited by stimulation of the sensory organs or peripheral nerves. It monitors the functional integrity of the pathways. However, it does not indicate the pathologic process or lesion involved. Evoked potentials (EPs) are small compared to the background EEG activity. Remarkably, evoked potentials are resistant to anaesthesia and sedative drugs. It is also resistant to the damage of the cerebral hemisphere unlike EEG. They are therefore used for monitoring the integrity of cerebral pathways in situations that render EEG useless. The interpretation of evoked potentials is based on certain factors. These are the prolongation of the latencies of the waveforms after the stimulus, the inter wave latencies and the asymmetries of the timing.

Visual evoked potentials (VEPs)

Visual evoked potentials (VEPs) are elicited by monocular (one eye after the other) stimulation. They are recorded from the occipital region in the midline and on either side of the scalp. There are three separate phases in the VEP waveform: an initial *negative* deflection (N70), a prominent *positive* deflection (P100), and a later *negative* deflection (N155). The P100 response is a signal at the midline occipital electrode which contains a prominent positive component and occurs approximately 100 ms after the pattern reversal. A delayed P100 in the full field VEPs of both eyes is frequently seen in demyelination. Other uses of VEPs include ocular abnormalities. This could be optic nerve disease (optic neuritis) from ischemia or compression by a tumor. Flash-elicited VEPs may be normal in patients with cortical blindness.

Brainstem auditory evoked potentials (BAEPs)

These are elicited by a single stimulation of the ear monaural (one ear after the other) with repetitive clicks (1000 to 2000) and are recorded between the vertex of the scalp and the mastoid process or ear lobe. They are helpful in screening for acoustic neuromas, brainstem pathology and the evaluation of comatose patients. The

BAEPs are normal in coma due to metabolic and toxic disorders or bilateral hemispheric disease. They are abnormal in the presence of brainstem pathology. A series of potentials, designated by roman numerals, occurs in the first 10 ms after the stimulus and represents in part the sequential activation of different structures in the pathway between the auditory nerve (wave I) and the inferior colliculus (wave V) in the midbrain. The presence, latency, and inter peak latency of the first five positive potentials recorded at the vertex are evaluated.

Somatosensory evoked potentials (SEPs)
These are recorded over the scalp and spine in response to electrical stimulation of a peripheral nerve. They are used to evaluate proximal portions of the peripheral nervous system. These are usually inaccessible. They also evaluate the integrity if the central Somatosensory pathways.

Clinical use of the sensory evoked potentials
Somatosensory evoked potentials may detect and localize lesions in the afferent pathways in the central nervous system. They are used to investigate lesions with multiple sites. Topmost on the list is multiple sclerosis in which the diagnosis requires the recognition of lesions involving several different regions of the central white matter. Others are AIDS, Lyme disease, Systemic lupus erythemathosus, Neurosyphillis, Spinocerebellar degeneration, Vitamins B and E deficiencies. The evoked potentials are sometimes used in prognostication in coma. Bilateral loss of the components generated in the cerebral cortex may imply that cognition may not be regained in posttraumatic or post anoxic coma. Preserved BAEPs in coma suggest a metabolic or toxic etiology.

17.30 Event Related Potentials
Event-related potentials (ERPs) are very small voltages generated in the brain structures in response to specific events or stimuli. Event-related potentials can be elicited by different sensory, cognitive or motor events. They provide safe and non invasive approach to study psycho physiological correlates of mental processes. ERPs are divided into 2 categories; early and later. The

early waves, or components peaking roughly within the first 100 milliseconds after stimulus, are termed 'sensory' or 'exogenous'. This is because they depend largely on the physical parameters of the stimulus. In contrast, ERPs generated in later parts reflect the manner in which the subject evaluates the stimulus and are termed 'cognitive' or 'endogenous' ERPs: they examine information processing. The waveforms are described according to latency and amplitude. The prolongation of the latency is seen in aging, dementia and other degenerative diseases such as Parkinson disease, progressive supranuclear palsy, and Huntington chorea. The amplitude is reduced in schizophrenia and depression.

17.40 Electromyography (EMG)
Electromyography evaluates and the records the electrical activity in the skeletal muscles. An electromyograph detects the electric potential generated by muscle cells when electrically or neurologically activated.

17.41 Uses of EMG
1. The EMG is commonly used in the diagnosis neuromuscular and muscles diseases
2. It is also used as a research tool for studying kinesiology, and disorders of motor control.
3. Recently, the EMG signals are sometimes used to guide botulinum toxin or phenol injections into muscles.
4. Other uses include the control of prosthetic limbs and monitoring of general anaesthesia with neuromuscular blockers.

17.42 Procedure
A pulse of electric current is applied to the skin, near the point of entrance of the muscular nerve (motor point). The required electrical pulse is brief, less than a millisecond, and is most effectively induced by a rapidly alternating (faradic) current. The pattern both at rest and activity are recorded from this needle electrode. Usually, relaxed muscles are electrically silent except in the endplate region. Spontaneous muscular activity is seen in various neuromuscular disorders. This is especially seen in those with denervation and inflammation of the muscle. The EMG is

usually performed with nerve conduction studies (NCS) except in cases of some purely primary myopathic conditions.

17.43 Abnormal patterns

Fibrillation potentials and positive sharp waves
Fibrillation potentials and sharp waves reflect muscle fiber irritability. They are usually found in denervated muscles, after muscle injury and in some inflammatory myopathic disorders like polymyositis. They may be persistent except renervation occurs or the muscle degenerates completely such that no viable tissue remains. In acute neuropathic injuries, they are found earlier in the proximal than in the distal muscles.

Single fiber electromyography
This is mainly used in detecting disorders of the neuromuscular junction. A special needle electrode is placed within a muscle. It is positioned to record action potentials from two muscle fibers belonging to the same motor unit. It is more sensitive than repetitive nerve stimulation and detection of acetylcholine receptor antibodies in the diagnosis of Myasthenia gravis.

17.50 Nerve Conduction Studies (NCS)
This is the main laboratory technique for the study of peripheral nerve. It is a complement the EMG examination. Needle EMG and NCSs are typically indicated when there is pain in the limbs, weakness from spinal nerve compression, or neurologic injury.

17.51 Uses of NCS

1. Nerve conduction studies are helpful in determining the level of the lesion: proximal or distal to the dorsal root ganglia. The peripheral sensory conduction will be normal in proximal lesions.
2. They are invaluable in localizing the lesion in mononeuropathies (compression or injury).

3. They are used to differentiate between mononeuritis multiplex and distal symmetrical polyneuropathies.
4. It is also used in monitoring progression and prognosis or peripheral nerve disorders

Spinal nerve injury does not cause neck, mid back pain or low back pain, and for this reason, evidence has not shown EMG or NCS to be helpful in diagnosing causes of axial lumbar pain, thoracic pain, or cervical spine pain.

References

1. Ekeh Bertha C; Clinical Neurology made Easy 1st Ed USA 2018
2. Epstein RJ. Medicine for examinations 4th Ed Canada 2006
3. https://en.wikipedia.org/wiki/Electromyography
4. https://www.ncbi.nlm.nih.gov/pmc/articles/PMC3016705/
5. https://en.wikipedia.org/wiki/Electroencephalography
6. Kasper DL, Fauci A S, Hauser S L, Longo D L, Jameson J L, Loscalzo J: Harrison's Principles of Internal Medicine; 19th Ed New York 2015
7. Lindsay K W. Bone I: Neurology and Neurosurgery Illustrated 4th Ed Edinburgh 2005
8. Ropper AH, Brown R H: Adams and Victor' Principles of Neurology 8th Ed New York 2005
9. Swash M, Glynn M: Hutchinson Clinical Methods 22nd Ed Edinburgh 2007

CHAPTER 18

TISSUE DIAGNOSIS

18.0 Introduction

Diagnosis in neurology may necessitate tissue biopsy with histology studies. The application of light, phase and electron microscopy to the study of samples from the brain, nerves, temporal artery, muscles and even the skin could be highly informative.

18.10 Stereotactic brain biopsy

Stereotactic brain biopsy is a procedure carried out by the neurosurgeon in the theatre. It involves mapping the brain in a three dimensional coordinate system. It entails the use of MRI and CT scans and 3D computer workstations to accurately target any area of the brain in stereotactic space (3D coordinate system). It is an important advancement in recent years. It exposes the patient to less risk than the craniotomy or open biopsy.

Indications
1. The main indication for stereotactic biopsy is in the diagnosis of deep-seated multiple lesions (especially suspected neoplasm).
2. Diagnosis of Creutzfeldt-Jakob disease (CJD) and some forms of viral encephalitis and granulomatous angiitis.
3. Definitive diagnosis of toxoplasmosis, tuberculoma, progressive multifocal leuco encephalopathy and cryptococcoma.
4. Surgically poor candidate who cannot tolerate anesthesia.

Technique
Stereotactic brain biopsy is a minimally invasive procedure. The procedure is carried out in the theatre under local anaesthesia by placing a head ring with four pins on the skull. Thereafter, a CT is performed. The patient also receives a light sedation. A thin biopsy needle is inserted into the brain using the coordinates obtained by

the computer workstation In most cases, the tissue sample is the brain; occasionally includes the scalp, blood vessels or the dura. Patients are monitored for several hours following the procedure and usually go home the same day.

Risks
The risks associated with stereotactic brain biopsy are minimal. Sometimes the sample of tissue obtained may be non-diagnostic, which may warrant a repeat biopsy.

18.20 Temporal Artery Biopsy
Superficial temporal artery biopsy (TAB) is the standard for making a diagnosis of temporal arteritis. It should actually be obtained almost without exception in patients in whom temporal arteritis is suspected clinically.

Procedure
In taken the biopsy, the correct selection of the site is important to improve yield and avoid complications. The focal symptoms like erythema, tenderness, jaw claudication and non pulsatile artery can help guide this selection. The artery is usually identified by visualization, palpation or Doppler USS. The artery usually biopsied is the frontal branch of the superficial temporal artery or the main trunk of the superficial temporal artery (when the frontal branch is atrophic). The recommended length is 2-5 cm of artery to provide accurate diagnosis of temporal arteritis since higher positive rates are noted with longer specimens. The use of longer specimens demonstrates the short, non contiguous foci of giant cell arteritis also called *skip areas*. Giant cells are seen on TAB in histology. TAB is a safe procedure; however, risks include temporary or permanent damage to the temporal branch of the facial nerve, infection, bleeding, hematoma, and dehiscence.

18.30 Muscle biopsy
This is an important step in establishing the final diagnosis of a myopathy. A specific diagnosis can be established in many disorders. It easily distinguishes the inflammatory myopathies as well as mitochondrial and metabolic myopathies. It is important to take the biopsy of the affected muscle to increase yield. In

inflammatory myopathies affecting the large proximal muscles, the muscle of choice for biopsy is the vastus lateralis of the quadriceps. Occasionally, the deltoid muscles may also be used. It should be noted that a biopsy should not be performed on a muscle that is very weak. This is because of the risk of picking an end-stage muscle where the lost myofibres have been replaced by fibro vascular and adipose tissue thereby masking the initial pathology.

18.40 Nerve biopsy

There are few indications that require this technique. A nerve biopsy may be taken at the ankle, forearm of rib. Nevertheless, the sural nerve at the ankle is the preferred choice for cutaneous biopsy. This is because the sural nerve does not supply any muscle. Nerve biopsy is discouraged in distal symmetric polyneuropathy because the yield is low. Indications for nerve biopsy include multifocal demyelinating neuropathies, vasculitis, leprosy, amyloidosis and sarcoidosis. It is also indicated when there is a palpable enlarged cutaneous nerve.

18.50 Skin Biopsy

The skin and conjunctiva are biopsied and examined in the diagnosis of storage diseases.

In choosing to perform a biopsy in clinical neurology, there are paramount issues to be considered. These include
1. Is there a likelihood of establishing the definitive diagnosis?
2. Will this diagnosis permit successful treatment or enhance management?

If these are not the case, biopsy is ill-advised because of its invasive nature.

18.60 Others

There are other specific investigations for diagnosis of neurological disorders. These are beyond the scope of this book.

18.61 Other Ancillary Investigations

Other investigations are carried out in neurological patients depending on the presentation. These are the full haematological profile, chemical pathology including hormone assays, toxicology screens and the microbiology including immunologic tests.

References

1. Ekeh Bertha C; Clinical Neurology made Easy 1st Ed USA 2018
2. Epstein RJ. Medicine for examinations 4th Ed. Canada 2006
3. https://www.ninds.nih.gov/Disorders/Patient-Caregiver-Education/Fact-Sheets/Neurological-Diagnostic-Tests-and-Procedures-Fact
4. https://emedicine.medscape.com/article/332483workup#
5. Kasper DL, Fauci A S, Hauser S L, Longo D L, Jameson J L, Loscalzo J: Harrison's Principles of Internal Medicine; 19th Ed New York 2015
6. Lindsay K W. Bone I: Neurology and Neurosurgery Illustrated 4th Ed Edinburgh 2005
7. Nwafor N N: Unpublished collections of Images
8 Rohkhamm R. Colour Atlas of Neurology 2ND Ed Stuttgart 2004
8. Ropper AH, Brown R H: Adams and Victor' Principles of Neurology 8th Ed New York 2005
9. Swash M, Glynn M: Hutchinson Clinical Methods 22nd Ed Edinburgh 2007
10. Walker HK, Hall WD, Hurst JW; Clinical Methods, The History, Physical, and Laboratory Examinations 3rd Ed Boston 1990

CHAPTER 19

GUIDE LINES TO INVESTIGATION

19.0 Introduction
The previous chapters have expounded the step wise process of localization of lesions. The importance of clinical evaluation comprising history taking and examination cannot be overemphasized. The clinical data guides to arrive at an anatomic localization thereby narrowing the differential diagnosis. Having identified the anatomical location of the lesion and identified the pathology and subsequent possible aetiology, relevant investigation is then carried out to confirm the clinical diagnosis. The investigations therefore may include may any of the following:

1. Laboratory investigation

a. Ancillary (Chemistry, haematology, microbiology, cytology and immunology)
b. Cerebrospinal fluid examination

2. Focused neuroimaging studies
3. Electro diagnostic studies
4. Tissue Diagnosis
5. Others

It has already been noted that some neurological disorders like tetanus, Rabies encephalitis and Parkinson disease do not require investigations for confirmation. This chapter therefore gives some guidelines based on the clinical features.

19.10 Investigations of the cerebral cortex

General pathologies in the cerebral cortex usually present with altered mental status, seizures or cognitive impairment. Other features are unilateral weakness, visual abnormalities and sensory abnormalities (including head and limbs) on one side of the body i.e. hemiparesis, hemianopia and hemianaesthesia.

Common pathologies in the adult patient include the following
1. Vascular: Cerebrovascular Infarcts, Intracerebral haemorrhage, SAH
2. Neurodegenerative; Alzheimer disease, Fronto temporal dementia, Dementia with Lewy Body
3. Infectious: Encephalitis, Cerebral abscess(various infectious agents
4. Neoplasia; Astrocytoma, Glioblastoma Multiforme
5. Intoxication
6. Trauma
7. Metabolic Disorders

The pathologies are either acute sub acute or chronic. They could also be generalized or localized. Vascular lesions, acute infections intoxication and trauma are usually acute in nature as already described.

Recommended investigations are as follows:

Brain Haemorrhage
Brain CT scan is the recommended investigation for all types of acute haemorrhage (intracerebral, intraventricular or SAH) is best seen on brain CT scan. This is because the CT scan visualises the haemorrhage which shows as a hyperdense lesion immediately. Sub acute haemorrhage and chronic haemorrhage are best visualized with brain MRI. CT scan may also be carried out (based on availability) however it is not very clear. In sub arachnoid haemorrhage, especially in suspected aneurysm, there is also need for CT or MRI Angiography to outline the intracranial vessels. Furthermore a lumbar puncture is required in suspected cases of SAH to differentiate it from Meningitis.

Ischaemic infarct
Traditionally, CT scan has been recommended as the first investigation to be carried out within 90 minutes of a cerebrovascular disease. The essence of this is to differentiate between haemorrhage and infarct. The infarct is not glaringly obvious until after 48-72 hours. Features of early infarct include loss of grey-white matter differentiation, Sulcal asymmetry, MCA sign and loss of attenuation. Currently, MRI with Diffusion (DWI)

which can detect the infarct within 10-20 minutes is the recommended as the first imaging procedure after an infarct.

However this may not be readily available especially in poor resource settings thus CT scan though limited remains the choice because of its availability. In haemorrhagic infarcts however, both CT scan and MRI are informative. Angiography (CT or MR) are required in all infarcts, carotid stenosis and vertebra basilar insufficiency. These cases also require Doppler USS to outline the vascular structures.

Suspected mass lesion
Mass lesions are usually not acute. They may be sub acute or chronic. They present with features of compression and raised intracranial pressure. Most of these are neoplastic lesions, infectious abscesses subdural haematoma. MRI with contrast enhancement is the required investigation of choice. In low resource settings, a CT scan with contrast enhancement is carried out because of the accessibility and cost considerations. These lesions will not be well visualized without contrast enhancement. In suspected vascular malformations like aneurysms, arteriovenous malformations; the required investigation is MRI with angiography. Some of these will also benefit from interventional procedures if available.

Generalized cerebral pathologies
Generalized lesions like seizures, sleep disorders and loss of consciousness usually require CT or MRI depending on the suspected aetiology since these are not diagnosis themselves. Common causes are infectious abscesses, haemorrhage and masses. Contrast enhancement is required in cases of infections and mass lesions. Other important investigations will be the full sepsis profile, CSF analysis, metabolic profile and toxicology screens. Hypoxic-ischaemic lesions are detected with an MRI image. Electrophysiology tests like EEG and its derivatives are required in seizure disorders.

Involvement of the meninges
Meningeal disease is often infectious, neoplastic or chemical. The required imaging modality is CT or MRI with contrast which should be performed before the LP to rule out raised intracranial pressure. C.S.F. analysis is of paramount importance in meningeal diseases. Other investigations will include the ancillary tests like full blood count, electrolytes and body fluid cultures.

Others
Most other cerebral lesions will require neuro imaging. In most of these cases, the MRI is more sensitive than CT scans.
In the spectrum of idiopathic inflammatory demyelinating (IIDDs) multiple sclerosis (MS), neuromyelitis optica (NMO), and acute disseminated encephalomyelitis (ADEM), MRI is required in the diagnostic criteria. The para ventricular lesions are highlighted in T2W and also by the FLAIR. However, there is no single MRI feature that distinguishes ADEM from NMO, MS, and cerebrovascular disease. There is need for contrast in the MRI of these demyelinating diseases. The visual evoked potentials may be informative in person with optic features.

Trauma
In acute trauma, CT is the required imaging modality because it is the better imaging modality in the examination of bone lesions. It will therefore detect fractures as well as haemorrhage, contusion and shear injury.

19.20 Investigation of the basal ganglia

Basal ganglia lesions present with abnormal movements hence, they are generally referred to as movement disorders. In most cases are bilateral like Parkinson disease and Huntington chorea. They may also be unilateral. Common causes of unilateral basal ganglia include infarcts and haemorrhage. Other causes are Rasmussen encephalitis, hemiballismus or hemichorea. The haemorrhage may be easily detected by CT scan. However other lesions like infarcts, encephalitis are better viewed with MRI. Note that the structures in the basal ganglia may be calcified physiologically. This calcification of the basal ganglia can give a false impression of haemorrhage. Some of the disorders may require further Specific investigations like the CAG sequence gene in Huntington chorea.

19.30 Investigation of the Brainstem

The brain stem as earlier noted functions as a conduit for all the tracts. Brain stem lesions have diverse features. They classically present with "Crossed" weakness and sensory abnormalities of head and limbs, e.g., weakness of right face and left arm and leg. There are also associated cranial nerve abnormalities (single or multiple). Other important features are loss of consciousness and cardio respiratory disturbances.

The most common brain stem lesions are CVDs and mass lesions (infectious abscesses, aneurysms and tumours). Brain stem features are also common in patients with the idiopathic inflammatory demyelinating disorders (IIDDs) i.e. acute disseminated encephalomyelitis (ADEM), neuromyelitis optica (NMO), and multiple sclerosis (MS). In the investigation of the brain stem, once again, the MRI especially the T2W and FLAIR sequences are the recommended imaging modalities. A contrast is required in suspected mass lesions. VEPs may be needed also. Other investigations especially in the unconscious patient will be electrolytes, urea, creatinine, blood cultures and toxicology screens.

19.40 Investigations of the cerebellum

Lesions of the cerebellum are usually mass lesions (infectious abscesses, cysts, tumours). They are best investigated with MRI which visualizes the structure: CT scan does not visualize the posterior fossa well. However, in poor resource setting, the CT may be the only available neuroimaging modality.

19.50 Investigations of the Spine and Spinal cord

The spine X-ray is an important cheap imaging modality in cases of trauma, abnormal curvature of the spine (scoliosis and kyphosis) and low back pain. The plain radiograph may reveal fractures, feature of degenerative disease, bone erosions and para vertebral abscesses. CT scan gives more information in investigation of the spine however; the scope of the scan is limited to the bone marrow. Lesions involving the spinal cord, conus medullaris, cauda equina and the nerve roots will require further evaluation with the MRI.

19.60 Investigation of the Peripheral Nerves

The peripheral nervous system involves both the cranial nerves and the spinal nerves. Cranial nerve disorders are usually part of the disorders of the cerebral cortex or brain stem and are investigated along.

Lesions of the spinal nerves cause weakness or sensory abnormalities following the nerve distribution. There may be "Glove and Stocking" distribution of sensory loss in distal symmetric polyneuropathy with associated loss of reflexes (initially the ankle jerk). Diverse nerves may be involved in mononeuritis multiplex. Common pathologies are metabolic, toxic and inflammatory conditions. Specific investigations of the spinal nerves will include nerve conduction studies usually in consonance with EMG. A nerve biopsy is necessary when multiple nerves are involved.

19.70 Investigation of the Neuromuscular junction and muscles

Neuromuscular junction disorders present with bilateral weakness (proximal myopathy) with early affectation of the head and neck muscles (ptosis, diplopia, dysphagia and snarl). There is associated fatigability (weakness with repeated use of muscles) with sparing of sensation.

Myopathies also present with bilateral proximal or distal weakness with sparing of sensation; however, they do not have the head and neck involvement. The weakness may follow a certain recognized pattern.

These lesions are investigated with EMG, NCS and in some cases, muscles biopsy. Other ancillary investigations may be carried out.

FURTHER READING

1. Baliga R R: 250 short cases in clinical Medicine 3rd Ed Saunders 2001.
2. Ekeh Bertha C; Clinical Neurology made Easy 1st Ed USA 2018
3. Epstein RJ. Medicine for examinations 4th Ed Canada 2006
4. Gates P. The Rule of 4s of the brainstem; a simplified method for understanding brainstem anatomy and brainstem vascular lesions for the non-neurologist Int Med J 2005; 35: 263-266
4. Harold Ellis: Clinical Anatomy 11th Ed Oxford 2006
5. Howlett. Neurology in Africa Bergen, Norway 2012
6. Kasper DL, Fauci A S, Hauser S L, Longo D L, Jameson J L, Loscalzo J: Harrison's Principles of Internal Medicine; 19th Ed New York 2015
7. Lindsay K W. Bone I: Neurology and Neurosurgery Illustrated 4th Ed Edinburgh 2005
8Rohkhamm R. Colour Atlas of Neurology 2ND Ed Stuttgart 2004
9. Ropper AH, Brown R H: Adams and Victor' Principles of Neurology 8th Ed New York 2005
10. Swash M, Glynn M: Hutchinson Clinical Methods 22nd Ed Edinburgh 2007
11. Walker HK, Hall WD, Hurst JW; Clinical Methods, The History, Physical, and Laboratory Examinations 3rd Ed Boston 1990

INDEX

Abducens nerve	41, 130
Acalculia	59
Accessory nerve	42, 132
Achromatopsia	63
Acute	147
Adenohypophysis	12
ADHD	91
Adie's tonic pupil	129
A geste antagoniste	89
Agnosia	62
Agnostic alexia	63
Akathisia	95
Akinetic mutism	57
Akinetopsia	63
Alexia	58, 63
All the 'Ds'	100
Allodynia	122, 124
Alpha coma	213
Alpha waves	210
Alzheimer disease	7, 74
Amnesia	66
Amygdala	8
Anaesthesia	122, 124
Analgesia	122, 124
Angiogram/Angiograph	177
Angiography	176
Anhidrosis	126, 127
Anomic aphasia	56
Anopia	129
Anosmia	128
Anterior cerebral artery	22
Anterior inferior cerebellar artery	24
Anterior Spinal artery	24
Anterior Spinal artery syndrome	116
Anterior 2/3rd Syndrome	116
Anterior cerebellar tract	33
Anterograde amnesia	67
Anton syndrome	9, 128
Arachnoid	19
Aphasia	54-56
Aphemia	65
Apraxia	63
Apraxia of speech	65
Aprosodia	59

Archicerebellum	18, 105
Argyll-Robertson pupil	129
Arnold –Chiari malformation	108
Around the clock	117
Artery of cerebral haemorrhage	22
Arteriography	176
Ascending Reticular formation	17
Ascending Tract	33
Association fibres	3
Associated features	150
Asthenia	105, 137
Asynergy	105
Ataxia	105
Athetosis	84, 90
Attention Deficit Disorder	91
Auditory agnosia	57, 62
Auditory cortex	7
Auditory nerve	41
Autonomic functions	121
Autonomic nervous system	36, 43, 44
Autonomic neuropathy	122, 126
Back kneeing	137
BAEPs	215
Balint's syndrome	61
Basal ganglia	10, 81, 230
Basal ganglia circuits	81
Basal nuclei	10, 81
Basilar artery	22
Basilar Pons	15
BBB	26
Becker muscular Dystrophy	138
Benedikt's syndrome	101
Beta waves	211
Bilateral ballismus	93
Binocular blindness	128
Bitemporal hemianopia	129
Bladder dysfunction	110
Blepharospasm	90
Blindness	128
Blood Brain Barrier	26
Bowel dysfunction	110
Brachial plexus	43
Brachial plexopathy	134
Bradykinesia	84
Brain stem lesions	96-104, 230
Brainstem evoked potentials	215

Brainstem herniation	104
Broca's speech area	5, 55
Broca's aphasia	55
Brown-Sequard Syndrome	115
Buccofacial apraxia	65
Bulbospinal tracts	10
Calcarine sulcus	8
CAT scan	181
Cauda equina	30
Cauda Equina syndrome	114
Caudal prefrontal cortex	6
Caudate nucleus	10
Cavernous sinus	25
Cavernous sinus thrombosis	25, 133
CECT	185
Central cord syndrome	116
Central sulcus	4,6
Central sulcus of Rolando	4
Cerebellar ataxic gait	105
Cerebellar lesions	105-108,230
Cerebellum	17
Cerebral cortex	2, 3
Cerebral peduncles	15
Cerebral venous system	25
Cerebrospinal fluid (C.S.F.)	20
Cerebrum	2
Cervical spinal nerves	43
Chiasmatic cistern	19
Chief Sensory nucleus	40
Chorea	84, 93
Chorea gravidarum	93
Choroid vein	25
Circle of Willis	21
Circumlocutions	56
Circumventricular organs	26,185
Cisterna ambiens	20
Chronic lesions	148
Cisterna magna	20
Cisterna pontis	20
Cisterns	20
Claude's syndrome	102
Claustrum	10
Colour anomia	58
Commissural fibres	3
Common carotid artery	22
Complete cord transverse lesion	115

Compressive cord lesions	107,118
Computerized Tomography	181-193
Conduction Aphasia	56
Confabulation	67
Coning	104
Conus medullaris	30
Conus medullaris lesions	114
Contrast Enhancement	186,187
Construction apraxia	65
Corpora Quadrigemini	14, 18
Cortical blindness	128
Corticospinal tract	33, 97
Craniopharyngioma	12
Craniosacral out flow	45
Crossed aphasia	55
Crossed paralysis	77
Cribiform plate	38
Crossed motor tract	33
Crural paresis	117
C.S.F. Analysis	155—171
C.S.F Appearance	160
C.S.F. Cellularity	162, 166
C.S.F. Chemistry	162
C.S.F Colour	160
C.S.F Culture	170
C.S.F Cytology	171
C.S.F Glucose	165
C.S.F Glutamine	166
C.S.F Lactate	165
C.S.F. Immunology test	170
C.S.F Microscopy	166-168
C.S.F Oligoclonal bands	164
C.S.F Pressure	160
C.S.F Protein	162
C.S.F. Transferrin	164
CT Index	185
CT scans	181-193
Declarative memory	74
Delta waves	211
Diaphragma sellae	19
Diencephalon	11
Diffuse lesions	144
Diffuse weighted imaging	199
Digit span	72
Digital subtracting angiography	177,178
Diploic veins	25

Diplopia	130
Direct pathway	82
Direct pyramidal tract	33
Dissociated anaesthesia	116
Dissociative amnesia	68
Dissociative fugue`	68
Distal symmetric polyneuropathy	143
Distal weakness	138
DMD	138 139
Divergent squint `	129
Dominant hemisphere	2
Dopaminergic	81, 82, 83
Doppler Ultrasonography	180
Dorsal pons	16
Dominant Hemisphere	2
Dorsolateral prefrontal cortex	6
Dressing apraxia	65
DSA	177, 178
Duchenne muscular dystrophy	138,139
Duck like	137
Dura	19
Duplex ultrasonography	180
DWI	199
Dysacusis	100, 137
Dysaesthesia	122,123
Dysarthria	106
Dyschronometria	105
Dysdiadokinesia	106
Dysgraphia	59
Dyslexia	58, 62
Dysmetria	61,107
Dysphagia	100,136
Dysphonia	100,136
Dystonia	84, 89, 90
Dystonic tremors	89
Echolalia	57
EC-Para hippocampus	7
Echo planar	200
Edinger- Westphal nucleus	39
EEG	206
Electro cerebral inactivity	213
Electro cerebral silence	213
Electroencephalography	206
Electromyography	217
EMG	217
Emissary veins	25

Enteric nervous system	46
Entorhinal cortex	8
Episodic memory	74
ERPs	215, 216
Event related potentials	215, 216
Evoked Potentials	214
Executive function	75
Extinction	62
Extradural cord lesion	111, 118
Extramedullary cord lesion	111, 117
Extrapyramidal disorders	83
Extrapyramidal lesions	83
Extrapyramidal motor system	10
Extra striate cortex	8
Facial nerve	41, 131
Falx cerebelli``	19
Falx cerebri	19
Fasciculus cuneatus	16
Fasciculus gracilis	16
Fast decaying memory	71
Fatigability	136, 137
Feed and breed	45
FEF	5
Fibrillation potentials	218
Fight or flight	44
Finger anomia	60
Flaccid paralysis	78
FLAIR	196
Floculo nodulular lobe	18
Fluid Attenuation Inversion Recovery	196
Foramen magnum syndrome	116
Foville's syndrome	102
Frontal abulic syndrome	69
Frontal disinhibition syndrome	69
Frontal Association Cortex	6
Frontal eye fields	5
Frontal lobe	4
Fugue state	68
GABAergic	81, 82, 83
Gait apraxia	65
Generalized cortical lesions	76, 228
Genu-recurvatum	137
Gerstamnn syndrome	61
Global aphasia	56
Globus pallidus	10
Globus Pallidus externa (GPe)	82, 83

Globus Pallidus interna (GPe)	82, 83
Glossopharyngeal nerve	41, 132
Glutamatergic	81, 82, 83
Glycorrhachia	165
Gradenigo syndrome	130
Gradient Echo	198
Gray matter	3
Great cerebral vein	25
Gustatory sweating	127
Headaches	77
Hemianopia	129
Hemi ballismus	93
Hemineglect	60
Hippocampus	8
Holmes –Adies pupil	129
Holmes rebound phenomenon	106
Homonymous hemianopia	129
Horizontal level	100
Horner's syndrome	99, 126
Hounsfield unit	184, 185
Huntington chorea	93
Hyperaesthesia	122, 123
Hyperalgesia	122, 124
Hyperdense	185, 190
Hyperhidrosis	127
Hyperkinetic disorders	83, 84, and 88
Hypermetria	105
Hyperpathia	122, 123
Hypnic jerks	92
Hypoaesthesia	122, 123
Hypoalgesia	122, 123
Hypodense	185, 190
Hypoglossal nerve	42, 132
Hypokinetic disorders	83, 84, and 85
Hypoglycorrhachia	165
Hypometria	105
Hypophysis cerebri	12
Hypothalamus	11
Hypotonia	105
Hypsarrhythmia	213
Hysterical tremors	87
Ideational apraxia	64
Identify pathology	145
Ideomotor apraxia	64
Immediate memory	72
Implicit memory	68

Indirect pathway	83
Inferior colliculus	14, 15
Inferior sagittal vein	25
Infratentorial	78
INO	98
Intention tremor	88, 108
Interbrain	11
Interictal epileptiform discharges	212
Internal carotid artery	22
Internal cerebral vein	24
Internal jugular vein	25
Internuclear ophthalmoplegia	98
Interpeduncular cistern	19
Interventional Angiography	178
Intradural cord lesions	111, 118
Intramedullary cord lesion	111, 117
Isodense	185, 190
Isolation aphasia	57
Lateral and anterior spinothalamic tract	34
Lateral corticospinal tract	33
Lateral geniculate body	38
Lateral medullary syndrome	103
Lateral sulcus	4, 6, 7
Lateral vestibulo spinal	10
Left common carotid	22
Lentiform nucleus	10
Light-near dissociation	129
Limbic network	54, 66
Limb kinetic apraxia	65
Locked in syndrome	103
Long term memory	72, 73
Loss of consciousness	77
Loss of grey-white matter differentiation	190
Lumbar cord lesions	113
Lumbar plexopathy	134
Lumbar puncture	155-158
Lumbosacral plexus	43
Lymphatic drainage of the brain	28
Magnetic Resonance Angiography	201
Magnetic resonance imaging	193-202
Magnetic Resonance Spectroscopy	202
Main sensory nucleus	40
Mandibular nerve	40
Mapping	143
Maxillary nerve	40
Medial lemniscus	14, 97

Medial longitudinal fasciculus	14, 97
Medial medullary syndrome	104
Medial prefrontal cortex	6
Medulla oblongata	16
Medullary pyramids	16
Memory	70-74, 107
Meninges	19, 219
Mesencephalic nucleus	40
Middle cerebral artery	23
Midbrain	14
Mid line shift	192
Millard-Gubler syndrome	102
Mixed dense	185, 190
Monocular blindness	128
Mononeuritis multiplex	143
Mononeuropathy	125, 143
Motor agnosia	63
Motor cortex	5
Motor neuropathy	125
Motor nuclei and nerves	98
Motor pathway	97
Movement disorders	10
MRA	201
MRI	193-202
MRS	202
Multifocal process	143, 144
Multiple cranial nerve palsies	133
Multiple lesions on CT	190
Multiple sclerosis	144
Muscle biopsy	223
Myasthenia gravis	136
Myelography	203
Myoclonic seizures	92
Myoclonus	92
Myokymia	91
Myopathic gait	137, 138
Myopathies	137
NCS	218
Nanotechnology	28
Negative myoclonus	92
Negative phenomenon	122, 124
Negative symptoms	149
Neocerebellum	18, 105
Nerve conduction studies	218, 219
Nerve biopsy	223
Neuromuscular junction lesions	136, 231

Neurohypophysis	12
Nigro –Striatal pathway	83, 84
Non compressive cord lesions	107, 119
Non Declarative memory	74
No-No tremor	89
Nothnagel's syndrome	101
Nucleus ambiguous	42
Nuclear magnetic resonance	193
Nystagmus	107
Obsessive Compulsive Disorder	84
OCD	84
Occipital association cortex	9
Occipital lobe	8
Occipito frontal network	54
Occulomotor apraxia	61, 65
Occulomotor nerve	38, 129
Olfactory nerve	38, 128
Ophthalmic nerve	39
One and half syndrome	98
Optic ataxia	61, 107
Optic chiasma	38
Optic nerve	38, 128, 129
Oral Apraxia	65
Orbitofrontal prefrontal cortex	6
Orthostatic hypotension	126
Orthostatic tremor	88
Quenckenstedt's test	156
Paleocerebellum	18, 105
Parahippocampal gyrus	8
Paramagnetic enhancement	198
Paramedian pontine reticular formation	97
Paraphasias	56
Parasthesia	122, 123
Parasympathetic nervous system	45
Parietal Association Cortex	7
Parietal Cortex	6
Parietofrontal network	54, 60
Parieto-occipital cortex	6
Parieto-occipital sulcus	6
Parinaud's syndrome	102, 129
Parkinson Disease	84, 85
Patterns of cord lesion	114-118
Perfusion Weighted Imaging	200
Peripheral neuropathy tremors	89
Peripheral nerve lesions	120-134, 232
Peripheral nervous system	36

Perisylvian network	54
PET scan	202
Phase contrast	201
Phenomic paraphasias	56
Phonagnosia	62
Physiologic tremors	87
Pia	19, 29
Pill rolling	88
Pineal Gland	15
Pituitary gland	12
Plain radiographs	173
Plexopathy	134
Polyneuropathy	128
Pons	15
Pontine sensory nucleus	40
Pontine tegmentum	16
Post calcarine sulcus	8
Posterior cerebral artery	24
Posterior columns	34
Posterior communicating artery	22
Posterior inferior cerebellar Artery	24
Posterior Spinal Artery	24
Posterior spinocerebellar tract	34
Position Emission Tomography	202
Positive myoclonus	92
Positive phenomenon	122, 123
Positive symptoms	149
Post traumatic amnesia	68
Postural tremor	88
PPRF	97
Pragmatics	59
Prefrontal cortex	5, 6
Prefrontal network	54, 70
Premotor cortex	5
Primary nucleus	49
Primary somatosensory cortex	7
Primitive reflexes	75
Principal nucleus	40
Procedural memory	68, 74
Projection fibres	3
Prosody	58
Prosopagnosia	62
Proximal myopathy	136, 137
Psychogenic amnesia	68
Psychogenic fugue	68
Psychogenic tremor	87

Ptosis	127, 136
Pure word deafness	57, 62
Putamen	10
Pyramidal tract	33
Quadrigeminal cistern	20
Radio density	185
Radiofrequency pulse	194
Recent memory	72
Recurrent lesions	150
Red nucleus	10
Reference memory	72
Relaxation times	194, 195
Remote memory	72
Rest and digest response	45
Rest tremor	88
Reticular formation	10, 16, 17
Reticulospinal	10
Retrograde amnesia	67
RF Pulse	194, 195
Rhythmic hyperkinetic movements	89
Right common carotid	22
Rubral tremors	89
Rubrospinal	10, 15
Rules of 4	96, 97
Sacral cord lesions	114
Sacral plexopathy	134
Scanning speech	106
Secondary memory	72
Secondary symptoms	151
Sella turcica	12
Semantic memory	74
Seizures	76
Sensory evoked potentials	216
Sensory memory	71, 72
Sensory neuropathy	122-124
Sensory nucleus of trigeminal nerve	99
SEPs	216
Sexual dysfunction	110
Sharp waves	212
Short term memory	72
Simian Posture	85
Simultagnosia	61
Skin biopsy	223
Skull X-Rays	173
Somatic nervous system	36
Spastic paralysis	78

Spike and slow wave complex	212
Spikes	212
Spinal cord	2, 29
Spinal cord lesions	108-118, 231
Spinal nerves	42
Spinal trigeminal nucleus	40
Spin density weighted imaging	199
Spine investigation	231
Spine X-rays	175
Spin –Lattice	195
Spinocerebellar tract	14, 99
Spinothalamic tract	14, 99
Spin-Spin	195
Staccato speech	106
Stereotactic brain biopsy	221
Striate cortex	8
Stuttering	6
Sub acute lesions	148
Sub arachnoid space	19, 29
Subclavian artery	23
Subcortical aphasia	59
Subdural space	19, 29
Substantia Nigra (SNr)	11, 82, 83
Subthalamic nucleus (STN)	11, 82, 83
Summary of site of lesions	141, 142
Superficial veins	26
Superior cerebellar artery	24
Superior Cerebral artery	24
Superior colliculus	14
Superior sagittal vein	25
Supratentorial	78
Suspended anaesthesia	116
Sylvian fissure	6
Sympathetic chain	99
Sympathetic dyspraxia	63
Sympathetic nervous system	44
T1 Relaxation time	194, 195
T1 Weighted Images	195, 196
T2 Relaxation time	194, 195
T2 Weighted mages	195, 196
TAB	222
Tactile agnosia	62
Tandem walk	105
Tardive dyskinesia	94
Tectospinal	10
Tectum	10, 14

Tegmentum	14
Temporal artery biopsy	222
Temporal Association cortex	7
Temporal lobe	7
Thalamostriate vein	24
Thalamus	12
Theta waves	211
Thoracic cord lesions	112
Thoraco-lumbar out flow	44
Tics	91
Titubation	89
Tolosa –Hunt Syndrome	133
Torsion spasm	90
Tourette's syndrome	84
Transcranial colour Doppler	180
Transcranial Doppler	180
Transcortical aphasia	57
Transient global amnesia	68
Transverse vein	25
Traumatic C.S.F	161
Tremors	84, 87
Trigeminal nerve	39, 128
Triphasic waves	212
Trochlear nerve	39, 127
Ultrasonography	179
Uncinate	126
Uncrossed	27
Upper cervical cord lesions	112
Vagus nerve	42,132
Vein of Galen	24
Venogram	178
Ventral tegmentum	14
Ventricular system	19
Ventrolateral prefrontal cortex	6
VEPs	215
Vermis	18
Vertebral artery	24
Vertical axis	101
Vestibulocochlear nerve	41, 129
Vestibular nucleus	10
Vestibulocerebellum	18
Vestibulospinal	10
Visceral nervous system	43
Visual associative agnosia	62
Visual agnosia	62
Visual Apperceptive agnosia	62

Visual cortex	9
Visual Evoked potentials	215
Visual object agnosia	62
Vocal tics	91
Waddling gait	137
Wallenberg syndrome	18, 103
Wall eyes	98
Weakness	77, 136-139
Weber's syndrome	99
Webino syndrome	98
Wernicke's area	54
Wernicke's aphasia	55
Wing beaten tremor	107
White matter	2, 3
Xanthochromic C.S.F.	163
X-Rays	173

Fundamentals of Neurological Diagnosis

Fundamentals of Neurological Diagnosis

www.ingramcontent.com/pod-product-compliance
Lightning Source LLC
Chambersburg PA
CBHW072132170526
45158CB00004BA/1346